Motivation, Sinn und Spiritual Care

Studies in Spiritual Care

Edited by
Simon Peng-Keller, Eckhard Frick,
Christina Puchalski and John Swinton

Volume 9

Motivation, Sinn und Spiritual Care

Herausgegeben von
Godehard Brüntrup und Eckhard Frick

DE GRUYTER

ISBN 978-3-11-078687-3
e-ISBN (PDF) 978-3-11-078715-3
e-ISBN (EPUB) 978-3-11-078720-7
ISSN 2511-8838

Library of Congress Control Number: 2022940988

Bibliografische Information der Deutschen Nationalbibliothek
Die Deutsche Nationalbibliothek verzeichnet diese Publikation in der Deutschen Nationalbibliografie; detaillierte bibliografische Daten sind im Internet über http://dnb.dnb.de abrufbar.

Printing: CPI books GmbH, Leck

www.degruyter.com

Inhalt

Godehard Brüntrup, Eckhard Frick

Motivation, Sinn und Spiritual Care

Die ersten Umrisse eines Spannungsfeldes

Die Aufsätze in diesem Band sind in einer interdisziplinären Fachtagung zu dem Thema „Motivation und Sinn" entstanden, die sowohl empirisch-psychologische als auch begrifflich-philosophische Zugänge eröffnen wollte. Auf den ersten Blick ist es aber alles andere als klar, welches der Zusammenhang von Motivation und Sinn ist, der hier untersucht werden soll. Nicht alles, wozu wir motiviert sind, ist sinnvoll. Nicht zu allem Sinnvollen sind wir motiviert. Begrifflich haben wir es mit einer Vielzahl von Bedeutungsnuancen zu tun. Unter „Sinn" verstehen wir sowohl die subjektiv erlebte Sinnstiftung als auch die objektiv zugemessene Sinnhaftigkeit. Das Eine ist ein mentaler Zustand wie „glücklich", das andere eine Werteigenschaft wie „gut". Der Begriff „Motivation" ist zunächst ein Konstrukt, das sich ganz allgemein auf die Bereitschaft bezieht, Anstrengung, Zeit und Energie für die Verfolgung eines Zieles einzusetzen. Abgesetzt wird die Motivation vom Willen, der dann eingesetzt wird, wenn es einen Mangel an Motivation bei der Verfolgung eines Zieles gibt. In der psychologischen Literatur werden vorwiegend drei Hauptmotive genannt, die alters- und kulturübergreifend anzutreffen sind. Da ist zunächst das Machtmotiv, also das Verlangen, sein Leben aktiv gestalten zu können. Positiv gewendet könnte man auch vom „Autonomiemotiv" sprechen, also der inneren Tendenz, das Leben so zu gestalten, dass man möglichst frei ist von äußeren Begrenzungen des freien Selbstseins. Das zweite Hauptmotiv ist das Bedürfnis nach Leistung und Kompetenz. Dem Menschen wohnt eine innere Tendenz inne, sich in der Bewältigung von Problemen und Aufgaben als fähig und geschickt zu erweisen. Das dritte Grundmotiv ist unser Verlangen nach Bezogenheit. Wir sind soziale Wesen, es motiviert uns, tun zu können, was unseren Bezugspersonen, unserer Familie und unserer Gemeinschaft zuträglich ist. Es motiviert uns, uns für etwas zu engagieren, das größer ist als wir selbst.

Ausgehend von diesen ersten Begriffsbestimmungen drängen sich nun aber schon Verbindungen von „Motivation" und „Sinn" auf: Sich für eine gerechtere Welt oder eine bessere Zukunft einzusetzen, ist etwas, das nicht nur sinnvoll ist, sondern auch als sinnstiftend erlebt werden kann. Man könnte sich zwar vorstellen, dass sich Mutter Theresa nur deshalb für die Armen eingesetzt hat, weil dies den ethischen Postulaten ihrer Religionsgemeinschaft entspricht. Aber das klänge merkwürdig und konstruiert, wenn sie ein solches Engagement nicht zugleich als etwas erleben würde, das ihren Bedürfnissen und Motiven entspräche,

https://doi.org/10.1515/9783110787153-001

zum Beispiel einem starken Bezogenheits- und Anschlussmotiv. Es mindert ihren heroischen Einsatz in keiner Weise, dass sie in ihrer Tätigkeit ein positives Gefühl der Bedürfnisbefriedigung empfindet. Wenn wir ein Ziel als sittlich geboten betrachten, dann ist es nicht allein durch diesen normativen Aspekt sinnstiftend, sondern auch weil die Verfolgung dieses Ziels eine natürliche Tendenz in uns, ein implizites gegebenes Ideal des guten Lebens, anspricht. Ein als sinnvoll erlebtes Leben ist ein solches, in dem wir uns mit dem beschäftigen können, was uns wirklich angeht. Man könnte im Sinne des Philosophen Harry Frankfurt sagen, dass die Verfolgung derjenigen Ziele, die uns wirklich wichtig sind („what we really care about"), eine Grundvoraussetzung für ein als sinnvoll erlebtes Leben darstellt.

Internalismus und Externalismus

Aber es bleibt die Frage, ob ein als sittlich gut erkanntes Ziel nicht auch ganz unabhängig von unseren angeborenen Motivkonstellationen aus sich heraus zum Handeln anstiftet und ob die Frage, ob wir ein sinnvolles Leben führen, begrifflich ganz unabhängig davon ist, welche inneren Bedürfnisse und Antriebe wir verspüren. Wir berühren hier eine klassische Frage der philosophischen Moralpsychologie: die Unterscheidung von Internalismus und Externalismus bei der Handlungsmotivation. Motiviert ein rein verstandesmäßig als gut erkanntes Ziel bereits notwendig zum Handeln? Das ist die Auffassung des Internalismus. Der Externalismus behauptet, dass die Motivation zum moralischen Urteil von außen noch hinzukommen muss. Der Urteilsinternalismus behauptet also, dass die Motivation schon innerhalb des moralischen Urteils liegt, dass also das moralische Urteil selbst motiviert, ohne dass ein begleitender Wunsch oder ein begleitendes Bedürfnis erforderlich ist. Ein Mensch, der nach seinen moralischen Urteilen lebt, ganz unabhängig davon, ob er auch den Wunsch zu einem solchen Leben verspürt, kann durchaus ein sinnvolles Leben führen. Nehmen wir als zuspitzendes Gedankenexperiment an, Mutter Theresa hätte eigentlich primär den Wunsch verspürt, ein hedonistisches Leben der unmittelbaren sinnlichen Bedürfnisbefriedigung zu leben. Die Vernunfteinsicht in das göttliche Gesetz wäre für sie bereits Motivation genug, ein aufopferungsvolles und entbehrungsreiches Leben im Einsatz für die Ärmsten der Armen. Aus internalistischer Sicht ist also die Einsicht in das moralische Gebot allein bereits motivierend, auch ohne stützende Bedürfnisse und Antriebe. Unstrittig ist, dass ein solches Leben sinnvoll ist. Es würde innerhalb aller großen ethischen Systeme als ein sinnvolles Leben angesehen werden. Können wir aber sagen, dass bei völliger Abwesenheit einer intrinsischen, bedürfnisbezogenen Motivation zu diesem Leben, die so konzipierte Mutter Theresa auch ein sinnerfülltes Leben führt? Kann ein als sinnvoll erlebtes Leben ohne jene Erfahrung des Glücks zustandekommen, die sich aus der Befriedigung eines mir innerlich gegebenen Antriebs speist? Diese philosophische Frage mag weltfremd und konstruiert wirken. Aus der Sicht der empirischen Forschung wird man fragen müssen, ob die hier vorausgesetzte strikte begriffliche Trennung von kognitiven Fähigkeiten einerseits und Emotionen und Bedürfnissen andererseits der Realität eines vernetzten neuronalen Systems entspricht. Ist die Trennung von Urteil und subjektiven Erleben, die Voraussetzung des Streites zwischen Internalisten und Externalisten ist, überhaupt sinnvoll? Zumindest auf eine kontingente Weise scheinen Vernunft und Gefühl in der Natur verbunden zu sein.

Der Urteilsinternalismus besagt, dass eine Person nicht aufrichtig ein moralisches Urteil fällen kann, ohne zumindest bis zu einem gewissen Grad motiviert zu sein, dieses Urteil auch in die Praxis umzusetzen. Die Einsicht in das Gute oder das Sinnvolle allein hat bereits bis zu einem gewissen Grad eine handlungsanbahnende Kraft. Der entscheidende Punkt liegt in „bis zu einem gewissen Grad". Die Erkenntnis, dass ein Einsatz für soziale Gerechtigkeit ein hohes moralisches Gut darstellt, motiviert, sich für dieses Gut zu engagieren. Aber es wäre eine rationalistische Verkürzung, der die westliche Philosophie seit Plato allerdings nicht selten anheimgefallen ist, zu meinen, rationale Einsicht und Schlussfolgerung allein motiviere schon *ausreichend* zum Handeln, wenn bloß die praktische Vernunft nicht beeinträchtigt ist. Das Phänomen der Willensschwäche ist gemäß dieser rationalistischen Tradition ein Defekt des Denkens: Man kann das, was als gut erkannt und damit gewollt wurde, aufgrund von Mängeln in der praktischen Vernunft nicht in konkrete Handlungen übersetzen. Alkoholgenuss könnte beispielweise die praktische Vernunft beeinträchtigen. Diese Analyse vermag aber nicht zu überzeugen: Willensschwäche ist vor allem darin begründet, dass man das für gut erkannte Ziel zwar „irgendwie schon", aber eben nicht stark und intensiv genug will. Willenschwäche ist ein motivationaler und nicht ein intellektueller Defekt. Man kann auch im Sinne der Existenzphilosophie sagen, dass das eine bloß rational erfasste Ziel zwar als sinnvoll erkannt wurde, es aber nicht innerlich sinnstiftend ist, weil es nicht *angeeignet* wurde. Es bleibt äußerlich, fremd und entfremdend, weil die Bindung an das eigene Selbst in seinem Ensemble von Wünschen, Bedürfnissen und Antrieben nicht gelang.

Die moderne Psychologie enthält implizit oft eine sehr schwache Form des Internalismus, also der These, dass die kognitive Erfassung eines Zieles allein schon motivierend sei. Das liegt darin begründet, dass man grundsätzlich zwei Zentren der Informationsverabeitung annimmt. Das eine ist bewusst, sprachlich und analytisch, das andere unbewusst, symbolisch und holistisch. In der Motivationspsychologie unterscheidet man dementsprechend zwischen expliziten und impliziten Motiven. Explizite Motive sind Ideale, Ziele und Projekte, die wir uns bewusst und in sprachlich verfasster Form setzen. Der bewusst gewählte Einsatz für die Gerechtigkeit durch ein Engagement bei *Amnesty International* wäre ein solches explizites Motiv. In diesem Sinne denkt die Psychologie also internalistisch: ein bewusst gesetztes Ziel hat bereits eine eigene motivationale Kraft. Aber diese Kraft ist schwach. Ohne Stütze durch entweder den Willen oder besser noch die impliziten Motive ist die Wirksamkeit der expliziten Motive sehr eingeschränkt. Auf den Schultern Freuds stehend anerkennt die Motivationspsychologie also, dass ohne die Unterstützung durch implizite Motive den expliziten Motiven oft die handlungsauslösende Energie fehlt. In diesem Sinne anerkennt sie die These des Externalismus. Wenn mein Ziel, bei *Amnesty International* für die soziale Gerechtigkeit zu arbeiten, beispielsweise durch ein starkes Anschlussmotiv unterstützt wird, dann verfüge ich über eine Energiequelle, die durch das explizite Denken allein nicht angezapft werden kann. Dieser soziale Einsatz ist dann nicht nur sinnvoll aus der Sicht einer rationalen ethischen Abwägung, sondern stiftet Sinn im Leben der handelnden Person, weil er ihrem Wesen, ihrem Selbst entspricht. Sie wird bei diesem Einsatz die emotional positiv gefärbte Erfahrung machen, etwas Sinnvolles zu tun, gerade weil diese Tätigkeit an eines oder mehrere ihrer Grundmotive angekoppelt ist. Ein starkes Leistungs- und Kompetenzmotiv wird ebenfalls die Ausdauer und Effektivität in diesem Einsatz erhöhen. Das wird wiederum dazu führen, dass die Tätigkeit nicht bloß sinnvoll ist, sondern als sinnvoll erlebt wird. Dieses Erlebnis der Sinnstiftung in der eigenen Existenz markiert einen wichtigen Zusammenhang zwischen Motivation und Sinn. Ohne die Aneignung eines als vernünftig erkannten Lebenssinnes als dem meinigen bleibt es bei äußerlichen und als fremdbestimmt erlebten Sinnvorgaben. Eine solche entfremdete Existenz kann nicht zu den positiven Affekten führen, die für ein sinnerfülltes Leben typisch sind.

Hat damit der Externalismus also doch den Sieg davongetragen? Ist Sinn dann eben nichts Objektives, sondern nur ein subjektives Sinnerleben, ein emotional positiv besetzter psychischer Zustand der Befriedigung. Damit sind primär nicht die einfach sinnlichen Bedürfnisse gemeint, sondern die tiefsten Sehnsüchte unseres Herzens. Ist Sinn also das Gefühl, das sich einstellt, wenn wir gemäß unserem „wahren Selbst" autonom und authentisch leben? Aber ist Sinn wirklich so subjektiv? Stellen wir uns einen Menschen vor, der seine Erfüllung darin findet, andere Menschen zu besiegen und auszuschalten und der sein Machtmotiv als starken Motor benutzt, um dieses Lebensprogramm authentisch und energetisch in die Tat umzusetzen. Ein solches Leben wird subjektiv als sinnstiftend erfahren. Von außen und aus einer objektiveren Perspektive erscheint vielen aber ein solcher Machthedonismus gerade nicht zu einem sinnvollen Leben zu führen.

Objektivismus und Subjektivismus

Dieser Frage nach dem Subjektivismus soll nun abschließend noch kurz nachgegangen werden: In der philosophischen Debatte um den Sinn des Lebens wird zwischen Subjektivismus und Objektivismus unterschieden. Der Objektivismus verortet den Sinn des Lebens in gewissen Zuständen der Welt. In einer gerechten Welt hat das Leben beispielsweise mehr Sinn als in einer ungerechten Welt. Die realisierte Idee der Gerechtigkeit ist also objektiv sinn-konstitutiv, weil die Idee selbst nichts rein Subjektives ist. Der Subjektivismus hingegen lässt den Sinn des Lebens von Mensch zu Mensch variieren, abhängig von den Einstellungen (pro-attitudes) des Einzelnen. Wenn Harry Frankfurt davon spricht, dass Fürsorge (caring) und Liebe (love) die Kriterien sind, nach denen der Lebenssinn gemessen wird, dann ist das eine Form des Subjektivismus. Denn jemand, dessen ganze Fürsorge und Liebe seiner Schallplattensammlung gilt, für den kann diese Sammlerexistenz der Sinn seines Lebens werden. Für jemanden, dessen ganze Fürsorge und Liebe ausschließlich seiner Familie gilt, kann es sinnvoll und sinnstiftend sein, die Interessen anderer Menschen rücksichtslos den Interessen der eigenen Familie unterzuordnen. Den meisten externen Beobachtern würden aber diese beiden Lebensentwürfe objektiv gesehen als wenig sinnvoll erscheinen. Fürsorge und Liebe, also Zustände der eigenen Psyche, können keine Garanten dafür sein, dass ein Leben objektiv sinnvoll ist. Das wirft nun eine interessante Frage auf: Führt die Kopplung von Sinn an den psychischen Zustand der Motivation notwendig zu einer subjektivistischen Konzeption von Sinn? Wenn Motivation auf subjektiven Bedürfnissen beruht und Sinn an Motivation gekoppelt ist, dann wird der Sinn selbst etwas Subjektives. Mit anderen Worten: Führt der Externalismus in der Moralpsychologie (ohne subjektives Bedürfnis keine Motivation) zu einem Subjektivismus in der Frage nach dem Lebenssinn (Sinn ist eine rein subjektive Sache)?

In der Psychologie selbst gibt es Gegenkräfte, die diesen Subjektivismus hinterfragen: Mit der „self-determination theory of motivation" der Motivationspsychologen Richard Ryan und Edward Deci kann man zwischen „integrierter Regulation" und „intrinsischer Regulation" unterscheiden. Integriert ist die Regulation dann, wenn das als sinnvoll betrachtete Ziel deshalb verfolgt wird, weil es in der Tat den tiefsten Bedürfnissen des eigenen Selbst entspricht. Im Sinne von Harry Frankfurt könnte man sagen: „What we really care about". Die erwähnte Selbstbestimmungstheorie der Motivation kennt aber mit der „intrinsischen Regulation" eine Form der Motivation, die erst dann erreicht wird, wenn eine Tätigkeit nicht nur deshalb als sinnvoll erlebt wird, weil sie den eigenen inneren Bedürfnissen entspricht, sondern weil die Tätigkeit selbstzwecklich als in sich sinnvoll betrachtet und erlebt wird. Die Freude an der Sache selbst kommt zur Freude an der Selbstverwirklichung noch hinzu. Beide gehören sogar zusammen. Man könnte es auch mit einem biblischen Paradox ausdrücken: Man gewinnt den eigenen Lebenssinn genau in dem Moment, wo man sich selbst nicht mehr ins Zentrum stellt, sich also in diesem Sinne „verliert". Wenn man eine Sache, die größer ist als man selbst, nur deshalb verfolgt, weil man ein inneres Bedürfnis hat dies zu tun, dann geht es einem noch nicht in reiner Form um die Sache selbst. Es gibt eine Form von Motivation, die erst dann wirken kann, wenn man sich ganz an etwas hingibt, das mehr ist als man selbst. Kein anderer hat diesen Gedanken stärker entfaltet als Viktor Frankl. Für ihn ist daher die Suche nach dem Sinn der größte Motivator. Sinnsuche ist der größte motivationale Antrieb. Setzt sich damit dann doch die rationalistisch-internalistische Konzeption durch, nach der allein die Sache selbst, die Idee und das Vernunfturteil motivieren? Verbinden sich rationalistischer Internalismus (die Idee allein motiviert) und Objektivismus des Sinns (Sinn ist nicht subjektiv) nun zu einer Einheit, welche die Bedeutung der subjektiven Wünsche und Bedürfnisse an den Rand drängt? Keineswegs: Das bloße Denken bleibt der ganzen Person immer äußerlich und kann gerade deshalb nur schwach motivieren. Sich einer Idee ganz hinzugeben, sich im besagten Sinne in ihr zu verlieren, ist viel mehr als die Idee nur mental zu repräsentieren. Ohne die bewusste Identifikation mit der Sache und die Integration der Ideen ins eigene Selbst bleiben die Ideale extern und fremd. Wir sprachen am Anfang davon, dass die Ideale „angeeignet" werden müssen. Vielleicht sollte man genauer von einer „aktiven Aneignung" sprechen, um den Unterschied zum bloßen Erlernen zu markieren. Die Wirksamkeit des Ideals hängt von der Aktivität des Subjektes ab, denn eine rein passive Teilhabe an der Idee wäre Fremdbestimmung. Es gibt aber auch Rezeptivität und Empfänglichkeit des Subjektes für etwas, das nicht aus ihm selbst stammt, in das es sich also verlieren kann. Im vollen Sinne ist man also motiviert, wenn man sich ein objektives Ideal aktiv subjektiv aneignet und sich von ihm zum Handeln anleiten lässt, weil man es an sich für sinnvoll hält. Dieses Zusammenspiel von subjektiver Aneignung und objektiver externer Wirklichkeit kann nicht auf die Seite des rein Subjektiven oder des rein Objektiven hin aufgelöst werden.

Spiritual Care?

Inwieweit können wir Harry Frankfurts Caring „spirituell" nennen? Der Doppelbegriff „Spiritual Care" stammt aus der Krankenbehandlung. Am bekanntesten ist Cicely Saunders' bio-psycho-sozio-spirituelles Modell von Palliative Care. Es wurde in offizielle Dokumente der Weltgesundheitsorganisation übernommen und wird inzwischen in vielen therapeutischen Kontexten verwendet.

Wird damit zur Begriffsliste somatisch / biologisch, psychisch, sozial ein weiteres Item hinzugefügt, ein weiteres To-Do für das therapeutische Team? Oder ist „spirituell" einfach ein wohltönendes Synonym für die externale Motivation, z. B. die ethischen Postulate der katholischen Kirche, die Mutter Theresa zum Engagement für die Armen motivierte? In ähnlicher (additiver) Weise wird oft auch die Berücksichtigung der Sinn-Dimension in Medizin, Pflege und Psychotherapie missverstanden: Als Perfektionierung der Krankheitsbewältigung durch Hinzufügen eines „meaning based copings", gewissermaßen als spiritueller Reservetank, wenn die problemlösenden und emotionsbezogenen Coping-Ressourcen erschöpft sind.

Die Gefahr des spirituellen Additionismus wird besonders deutlich am gegenwärtigen Resilienz-Diskurs: Der Resilienz-Begriff ist derartig normativ aufgeladen, dass er das spirituelle Feld in einer Leistungsethik aufsaugt: Verbundenheit (connectedness), Transzendenz, Sinn-Konstitution (meaning-making) werden zu Postulaten: Man muss spirituell sein, um seine Resilienz unter Beweis zu stellen, gerade unter Belastungsbedingungen (z. B. ökonomische, pandemische, klimatische oder Beziehungs-Krisen).

Angesichts der skizzierten Tendenz, die Spiritualität therapeutisch zu instrumentalisieren, sei auf das kritische Potenzial der Begriffe „spirituell" und „Spiritualität" hingewiesen. Schon die geistliche Tradition spricht von „Unterscheidung der Geister" und bietet differenzierte Kriteriologien des Wahrnehmens, des Wertprüfens und Handelns an, z. B. innerhalb der auf Ignatius von Loyola zurückgehenden „Spirituellen Übungen" (Exerzitien): Ignatius lehrt Regeln, um die das Subjekt bewegenden „Geister" und Spiritualitäten im Längsschnitt zu bewerten, nicht nur im Querschnitt der internalen oder externalen Momentaufnahme.

„Spiritual" als Epitheton zu „Caring" kann nur dann ein kritisches Potenzial entfalten, wenn Motivation und Sinnsuche im Horizont der Transzendenz gesehen werden: Transzendenz ist unzugänglich für unser Messen, Behandeln, Optimieren. Aber gerade die Unverfügbarkeit einer auf die Transzendenz verweisenden Spiritualität motiviert zum Handeln und zur Freiheit in den uns (innerhalb der Immanenz) gesetzten Grenzen.

Benjamin Andrae

The Purpose of Life

Die Sinne des Lebens

Zusammenfassung: Der Artikel untersucht die Frage nach dem Sinn des Lebens, wobei das Wort „Sinn" in der Bedeutung ‚Ziel, Zweck, Wert, der einer Sache innewohnt' (siehe: „Duden.de") verwendet wird. Als Antwort auf diese Frage wird ein realistisch verstandener, ausgedünnter Pluralismus als theoretische Position vorgestellt, die sechs mögliche Antworten bietet: Glück, Wahrheit, Moralität, Schönheit, Liebe und Demut. Besondere Aspekte der hier vorgestellten Position sind die folgenden zwei: Erstens sind laut ihr die Sinne eines individuellen Lebens nicht einfach alle diese genannten, sondern jede Person hat ihr eigenes „Mosaik" der Sinne des Lebens – geformt teilweise durch Zufall, teilweise durch Veranlagung und Prägung und teilweise durch fortlaufende Selbsterschaffung. Zweitens ist die Position durch einen nur moderaten epistemischen Anspruch gekennzeichnet – da sie als Resultat einer vier Jahre währenden Diskussion mit deutschen Gymnasiasten verstanden wird, und nicht als selbstevidente Wahrheit. Vier Argumente, die für diese Position sprechen, werden ins Feld geführt: Sie ist produktiv, sie vermeidet Despotismus, sie ist nicht von klassischen Gegenargumenten betroffen, die normalerweise gegen „objective-list theories of well-being" aufgeführt werden, und sie erlaubt, dass die Sinne des Lebens sich im Verlauf eines individuellen Lebens verändern.

Durch die Diskussion von ‚Ziel, Zweck, Wert, der dem Leben innewohnt' wird die oft auf Englisch gestellte Frage nach dem „meaning of life" nicht vollständig beantwortet, da diese eher nach dem semantischen Gehalt des Wortes „Leben" – also grob nach einem umfassenden Verständnis aller Aspekte des Lebens – zu fragen scheint. Allerdings ist mit einer Aussage über den Zweck des Lebens ein Teil des „Meaning of life" erklärt – und vielleicht sogar der Teil, der viele Fragende am meisten interessiert.

Schlüsselwörter: Sinn des Lebens, Gelungenes Leben, Selbst-Erschaffung

Abstract: A Realistically Understood Scarce Pluralism is presented as a theoretical position that answers the question "What is the purpose of life?" by naming six purposes: Happiness, Truth, Morality, Beauty, Love and Humility. The presented position is special in two senses: First, it includes the claim that the purposes of an individual life are not simply all or the possible ones, but an individual "mosaic" that owes its shape partly to chance, to nature and nurture, and to

https://doi.org/10.1515/9783110787153-002

continual self-creation. Second, it is only moderately epistemically ambitious, since it is considered the result of a four-year intelligent discussion with teenage students at a German high-school. Four arguments that speak for this position are presented: It is productive, it avoids despotism, it avoids classical criticisms of objective-list theories of well-being and it allows for flexibility during the course of a human life.

Keywords: Purpose of life, Meaning of life, Well-being, Self-creation

The question

"What is the purpose of life?" In this essay, I will present a theoretical philosophical position about how to answer this question. First, the focus will be on the form of the answer. In the next step, I will discuss how the purposes of life actually might manifest themselves in the life of an individual. Then, in the third step, the actual answer(s) that I suggest will be presented, albeit in a much-condensed form.

Before discussing the answer, though, we need to discuss the question: "What is the purpose of life?" As this question is understood here, it can also be formulated as "What goals should I try to reach in life?", "What are the values that I should try to incorporate into my life?" or simply "What are the things that make my life a *good* life?". The question about the purpose of life is a question about teleology, about the final causes of life.

Not only but also thanks to Monty Python, in the English-speaking world, the question "What is the *meaning* of life?" is much more common; hence, it will prove useful to point out overlaps and differences between this question and the one that I talk about in this essay. The first thing one notices is that the question about the meaning of life is very vague. If one puts the focus on the word "meaning", it seems to be a question about semantics. Yet, the things that usually have (semantic) meaning are words and sentences, and since life is neither, the question might not even be well-formulated. Unless, of course, it asks "What is the meaning of the word 'life'?" – a question to which the Merriam-Webster dictionary provides 20 different answers. More broadly speaking, though, we use the word "meaning" in the context of trying to understand something: A scientist might look at her results and ask: "But what does this mean?"; And a therapist might ask: "What does the dream mean to you?". Both these examples can be understood as the search for an interpretation, for a theory about something in the world. Hence, the question "What is the meaning of life" might be understood as an attempt to interpret life, to gain an encompassing theory of it. Such a theory would, presumably, amongst many other things also include a statement about the purpose of life. Thus, we can say that the question about the purposes of life is a partial answer to the question about the meaning of life.

Sometimes, everyday language even seems to put the purpose-aspect front and center: When we say "I finally found a meaningful job!", we usually do not mean that we found a job that we can interpret well, but we mean that we found a job that allows us to strive towards good goals, that incorporates values that we approve of, etc. And when we say "My life has lost all meaning", it might often be the case that we mean that there is nothing left in life that we feel would be worthwhile doing. This way of using the word "meaning" also seems to be the one that stands behind the commonly used English translation of Viktor Frankl, when he famously talks about "...meaning in life", which can be arrived at by "creating a work or doing a deed", by "experiencing something or encountering someone" or by changing oneself in hopeless external circumstances that one cannot change, thus turning "a personal tragedy into a triumph" (Frankl 1959: 145 f).

In these purpose-centric ways of using the word "meaning", the question about the meaning of life is just the same question as the one about the purpose of life.

Two background details

There are two background details for what follows that are not the main concern of this essay, but that are nevertheless important to mention: First, I will only talk about human life. The reason is that I assume that if one were to include animal life, the question would be much more difficult to answer than it already is. This limitation does not in any way mean that it is assumed that animal life does not have a purpose, or that it has purposes that are very much different from the ones I will be talking about for humans. On the contrary: For example, with great apes or dolphins, it intuitively seems like some of the things that can make their lives good are just the same as they are for us – they seem (to me) to be able to love, they seem (to me) to appreciate beauty and they seem (to me) to strive for happiness. But I am far less confident that this is really true, since it might also be a case of me projecting human categories on beings that should have their own categories.

The second background detail is a basic assumption that is necessary for the idea of a purposeful life in the sense of the purposes presented in section five to make sense, but that I will not argue for: It is taken for granted that a human life is not completely contained within the present, but also includes the past to some extent. This is important because it means that a life can be good, can fulfill its purpose, even if it does not do so *right now*. If I am usually very happy, but right now I am in great pain and not happy at all, my life is still a good life according to the purpose of life that is happiness. Or if I have spent my life in loving relationships, but now that I am old all my family and friends have died, my life can still be a good life according to the purpose of life that is love. Such a continued existence of the past of a human life also rules out the idea that life cannot have a purpose just because, as Bertrand Russell puts it, eventually "all the labours of the ages, all the devotion, all the inspiration, all the noonday brightness of human genius, are destined to extinction in the vast death of the solar system, and [...] the whole temple of Man's achievement must inevitably be buried beneath the debris of a universe in ruins" (Russell 1903: 47 f).

Taken to its philosophical conclusion, this way of thinking about the past would lead into deep metaphysical territory; but – just like the purpose of animal life – that will not be the topic of this essay.

The form of the answer

The position that I will present and argue for is a *Realistically Understood Scarce Pluralism* about the purposes of life. To explain what this means, the two aspects of this position will be described separately.

To say that the purposes of life should be *understood realistically* means that there are objective facts of the matter as to what makes my life good. Whether my life has purpose is not a matter of my personal mental state, especially not of my desires. Derek Parfit puts this by saying "Though it is good to have sensations that we like, nothing is good merely because we want this thing" (Parfit 2011a: 55).

Since, usually, it is assumed that I have some kind of control over my mental states – I can, for example, eventually overcome my desire for chocolate cookies –, but I have no control over these objective facts, this means that in this view I have no control over what the purposes of life are. Whether a given way of life has purpose is decided by the world, and not by me.

Now, saying that something is to be understood realistically leads to the question as to what exactly this entails ontologically. Here, we are presented with different options, all of which would work with the position outlined above. One such option – which in my view is preferable for reasons beyond the present topic – is Whitehead's "Civilized Universe" (Whitehead 1938, lecture 6): Whitehead argues that the whole universe, even the movement of electrons or the formation of galaxies, is in some way 'civilized' – by which he means that it is filled with and moved by values and ideals. This ontology directly connects to the human world, since – as David Ray Griffin puts it – it provides "a cosmology intended to support the ideals now needed by human civilization" (Griffin 2001: 287). Another option would be a "simple" Platonic metaphysics, in which the ideals that can make human life good exist eternally in a realm of ideas, which somehow interacts with concrete human life. What is important for this essay, though, is not the choice of ontology, but merely the fact that a sensible ontological interpretation of realistically understood purposes of life is possible.[1]

We will now move on to the second aspect of the position presented here: To say that there is a *scarce pluralism* of purposes of life simply means that, on the one hand, there is more than one purpose but, on the other hand, there is only some fairly small and definitely finite number of them; and that there is no explicit or implicit hierarchy of these different purposes – none of them is per se better or more important than all or some of the others. An excellent way of putting this is given by Parfit, when he discusses Frankfurt's position and presumes to describe Frankfurt's "real view" – which would be just such a scarce pluralism:

> When we are deciding how to live, Frankfurt also writes, we need to decide which of several possible ends we shall try to achieve. These ends include personal satisfaction, pleasure, glory, creativity, spiritual depth, and conformity with the requirements of morality. Frankfurt's list does not include personal dissatisfaction, pain, dishonor, futility, spiritual shallowness, and immorality. [...] On what seems to be Frankfurt's real view, there are many intrinsically good ends, but no ends have supreme value. Nor are there precise truths about which ends are most worth achieving. We often have to choose between many good ends or aims [...]. These plausible claims are very different from the view that no ends are in themselves good. Frankfurt, I suggest, is not a Nihilist about intrinsic goodness, but a Pluralist (Parfit 2011a: 55).

In the scarcity, there is a connection to the other aspect of the position presented here: It is only because in this position the realistically understood purposes do not depend on the mental states of humans, and thus are not under a subject's (partial) control, that we can hold that there is a small finite number of such pur-

1 Parfit seems to think that one does not even really need that because he thinks that truths about objective reasons "can be plausibly claimed to exist [...] also in a distinctive, non-ontological sense" (Parfit 2011b: 480). This way of speaking seems to be motivated by the view that distinct ontological implications somehow reduce the worth of a theory (see, for an example from the context of Parfit's theory, Mintz-Woo 2018) – whereas I, with Whitehead, would hold that eventually, every philosophical discussion reaches "a stage of thought for which metaphysics is essential to clarity" (Whitehead 1929: 146).

poses. If, on the other hand, purposes were determined by human choice, their number would be very difficult to keep small – because, given time, humans could probably be made, by themselves or others, to desire all sorts of things, be it the success of a certain sports team, the dominance of their nation over others or, to use Rawls' famous example, to know the exact number of blades of grass on the lawns of Harvard.

How an individual answer comes about

The first question that springs to mind upon hearing the position presented above is: "If there are (some) different purposes of life, do I need to attain them all?". This seems impossible, because how can you attain, say, the moral good of a life's work as a medical doctor, the aesthetic good of creating sublime works of art, the epistemological good of gaining a deep understanding about human nature, the interpersonal good of living in loving community with others while also having enough leisure to feel happy and stress-free at the same time? The main reason that this impossibility seems obvious is the fact that humans have limited time and energy. But there are also cases where these different purposes actively seem to contradict one another: Doctors might become less happy precisely because of the morally good work that they do that puts them in contact with a lot of human suffering; knowing too much might also decrease the chance at happiness ("Ignorance is bliss"), an analytical mindset might prove to be detrimental to the more intuitive ways of thinking that an artist employs, etc. I am not confident that any single one of these concrete examples is true, but the amount of such prima facie plausible examples makes me confident that there really are cases where different purposes actively contradict each other. Hence, because of both the limitation of time and energy and contradictions between purposes, I hold that it is impossible to attain all the purposes of a realistically understood scarce pluralism in one's own life.

This leads straight to a second question: "If there are more purposes to life than I can fulfill, then which are the purposes of my life?". The position I present here answers with a *part chance, part nature and nurture, part self-creation mosaic-view.*

"Mosaic-view" means that it is assumed that an individual can have more than one of the different available purposes of life, and that in each such individual mosaic these purposes can vary in strength: One person might strive for love and knowledge equally but not so much for acting morally; another person might value creating art very highly, also to some extent strive for happiness, and disregard the rest; a third person might only look for spiritual depth, and become a hermit – ignoring any other possible purpose of life.

"Part chance, part nature and nurture, part self-creation" means that how each individual mosaic is composed depends on three factors. First, chance plays a role: If by accident I do not meet other people that I get along with, it will be less likely that I spend my life in loving community with others, for example. Secondly, who I am – also with regards to the purposes of my life – is partially determined by my genes and my upbringing: If, as a result of either or both, I am less interested in learning, then it will be less likely that attaining knowledge becomes a central purpose of my life. And thirdly, I claim that there also is a certain way in which we make ourselves into the people that we become. While the first two factors are less likely to be contended, the third one is highly controversial – hence, in what follows, I will focus on this point. Self-creating is certainly not a mere matter of normal choice, since to really choose, you need a value that you already have that informs your choice: "I choose to go to the Italian restaurant tonight, because there I expect to be the happiest – and I want to be happy". If there is no such value, you do not choose, you just pick at random. But creating a new purpose of your life is a value-change, and thus it does not make sense to think about it as the way of thinking about normal choice. The idea of self-creation that the position presented here employs is that of "aspiration", as presented by Agnes Callard. She holds that a person is capable of "value-learning" (Callard 2018: 257) in a radical sense that is more than just self-improvement based on already present values, and more than just being shaped by chance or by circumstance: Agents, according to this view, can act for "proleptic reasons", i.e. reasons that lie in the future, for example when one wants to learn to appreciate classical music without doing so now.

> When we say that the aspirant's grasp is "proleptic", what we mean is that her grasp of the value for the sake of which she acts is a dimension in which she improves herself over the course of her aspirational agency. At the end of the process, she will be able to say, truthfully, "Now I see what I was after all along!" Did she grasp this end all along? Yes and no: she grasped it enough to be "after" it, but not enough to see it for what it really is (Callard 2018: 258).

These proleptic reasons lie in the future, but this does not mean that there is backwards causation in the sense that a future event is the effective cause of something that is happening now – there are plenty of past effective causes that can causally explain why I try to get into classical music. However, the normative reason why I do this *does* lie in the future. Callard says "My claim, then, is that in the case of aspiration, causal or temporal priority fails to track normative priority" (Callard 2018: 213).[2]

If one accepts that self-creation is a part of what constitutes an individual's mosaic of the purposes of life, as I do, then we have to revisit and specify something said above: While, on this position, one does not have control over what the purposes of life are (since they are objectively understood), one does have some control over which of these purposes are relevant for one's own individual life.

A third, related, question one might be inclined to ask in this context is: "How can I know which of these different purposes of life are in my mosaic? (Regardless of how they got there.)" Here, the position presented in this essay makes an important claim: *There is always some positivity in my own mental states that has the potential to tell me which purposes of life are "for me"*. This positivity does not have to be – but can be – a conscious, cognitive awareness of value, and it does not have to be – but can be – a feeling of great joy whenever I act in accordance with a purpose. It might also be a feeling of "this is right"-ness, or a sense of duty or an intuition that this is my calling, or an increase of peace of mind or an absence of a guilty conscience. Or it might be a clearness and absence of confusion. The example, from the description of "proleptic" reasons given above, of the person trying to learn to appreciate classical music is another good case: As long as I have no real clue about classical music, I cannot really say that the perception of beauty – in so far as it is contained in this appreciation of classical music – is one of my purposes of life. Because I do not know the value enough to perceive its "goodness". In this vein of thought, another mental state that might help me find out which of the purposes of life are really mine might be that of really knowing and understanding a purpose for the good that it is.

Amidst all these examples, I am not claiming that each and every one of them is suitable – some might very well be problematic. All I claim is that some positivity in my mental states can guide me towards finding out what my purposes are.[3] This claim has some interesting consequences: For example, it means that a true nihilist – someone who really, deep down, has no positivity about any purpose in any of their mental state, if that is possible – really has no purpose in life, at least not until they change substantially. It also would imply that someone who really has no conscience at all, and no other positive mental

2 Again, there is a lot left to be specified as to what this might mean in an ontological sense. And again, Whitehead's philosophy, especially his idea about the subject-superject (see Whitehead 1929: 222), might prove useful in this context.

3 Note that I do not claim that this will always work. I can certainly be wrong about my purposes of life, just like I can be wrong about many other of my mental states.

state about caring for others, does really not gain any purpose in their life if they – accidentally, I would presume – follow the requirements of morality.[4]

There is one more interesting aspect that I want to highlight in this context – because it will be relevant in the next section. As the examples for involved mental states already hinted at, getting to know one's purposes in life is a process that happens not only in clear, cognitive thought but heavily involves the unconscious mind. And one way to take this into account is to reflect upon the purposes of life using other faculties than just cognitive thought. Pictures and metaphors might prove especially useful to see what purposes resonate with me on a deep level. Godehard Brüntrup puts this as follows:

If one wants to harmonize unconscious basic motives with those of the second order that can be formulated in language, this will not work using language or thought, because in these cases the unconscious mind does not get involved. The common medium is rather pictures, metaphors (Brüntrup 2020, translated from German by Benjamin Andrae).

The content of the answer

A realistically understood scarce pluralism should be able to name at least some of the purposes of life. In this section, this is what I will do. In accordance to what was just said about the important role of the unconscious and how it can get involved, these will be presented as a set of pictures only. For a longer exposition of how one could conceive each of these purposes, focusing on how it would manifest itself in everyday life, choice of job etc., see Andrae (2018).

The method used to arrive at this set, though, is somewhat unusual: In addition to my mostly introspective armchair-reasoning – "self-evidently, these are things that make a life *good*..." – I have spent four years discussing the purposes of life with German teenagers between roughly the ages of 15 and 18 while teaching philosophy at a German school. In the course of discussions, some ideas that I had brought with me were modified or discarded, and some new ones were picked up. Hence, it can be said that the following set of purposes of life is somewhat a consensus between many different people – many of which were teenagers, who, in my experience, have a very serious attitude towards the question

4 If this seems wrong to you, as it does to me, one could simply make the claim – that seems right to me – that everyone has a conscience, however difficult circumstances have made it for many of us to listen to it.

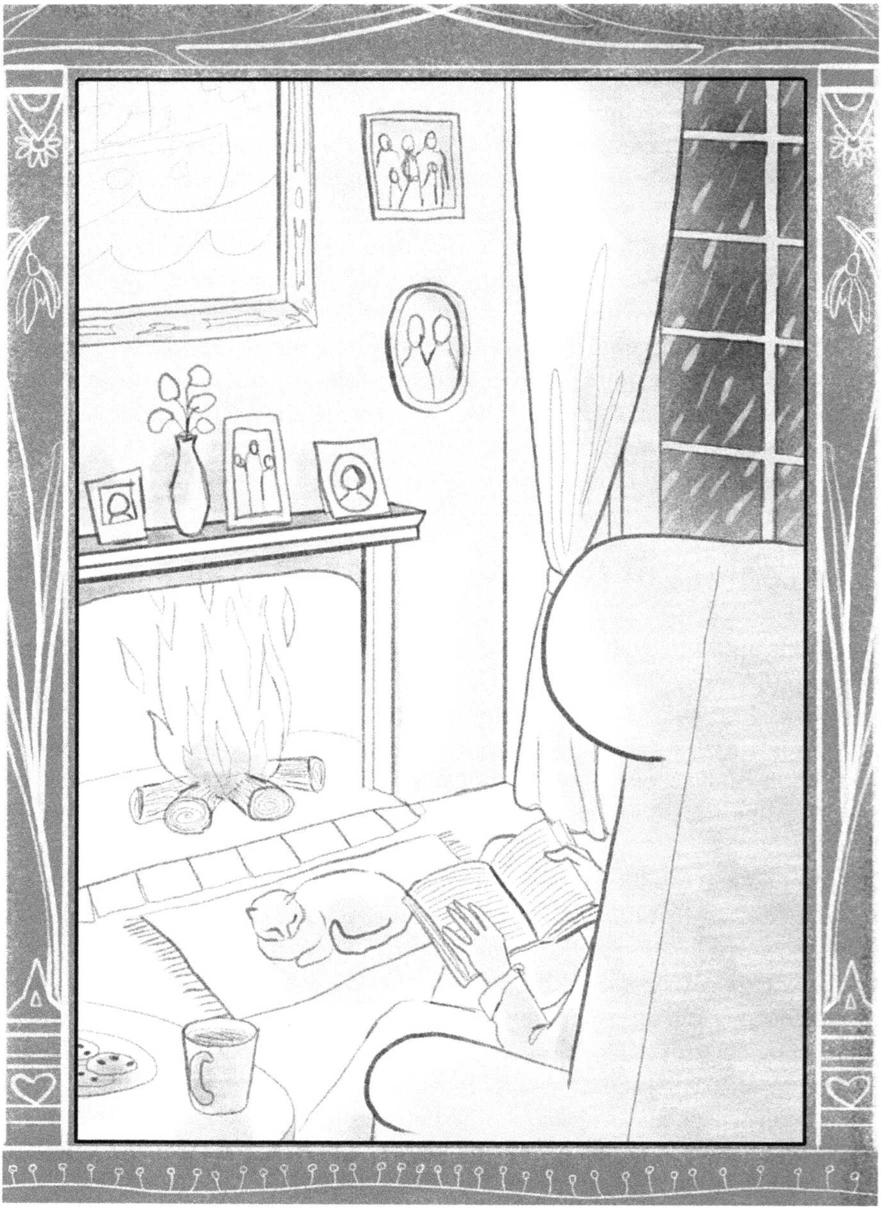

Figure 2.1 “Happiness” (Illustration: Caroline Hamann).

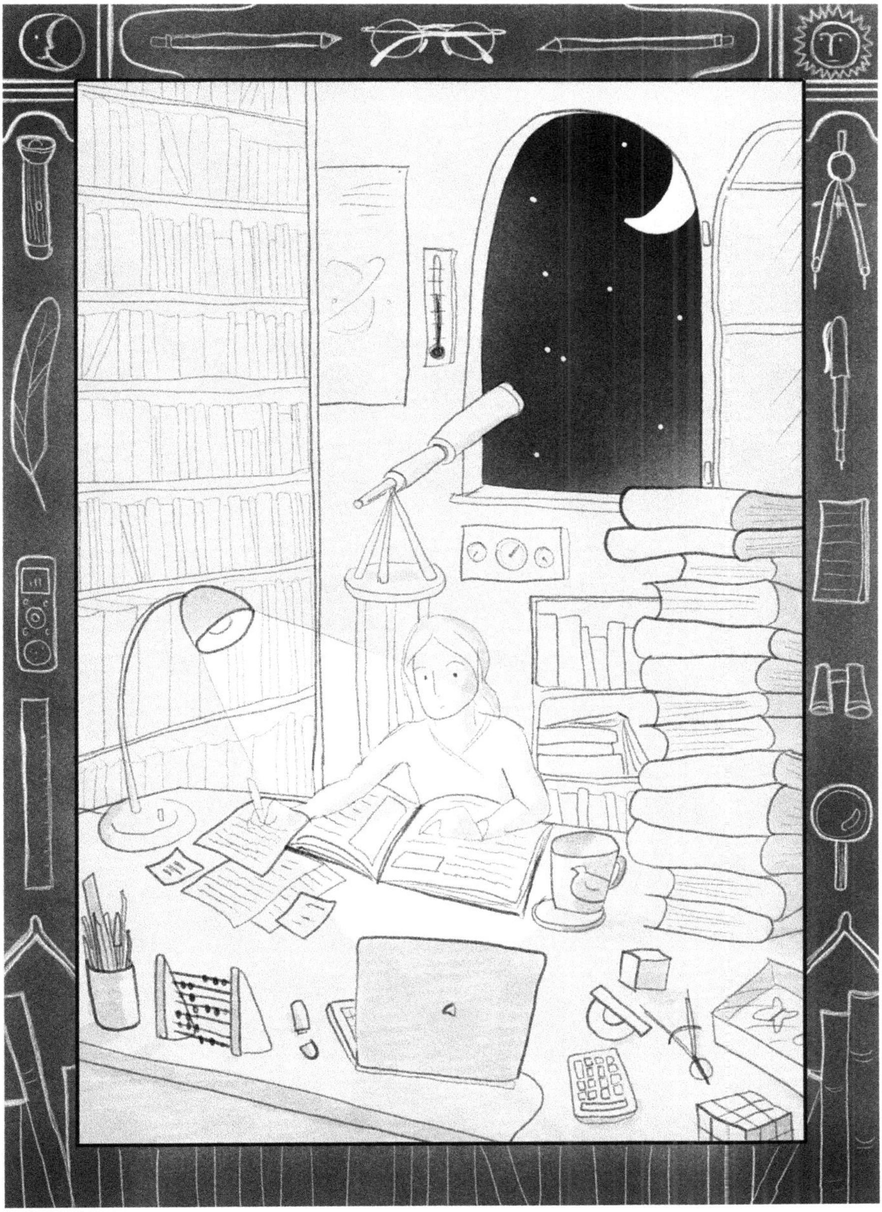

Figure 2.2 "Truth" (Illustration: Caroline Hamann).

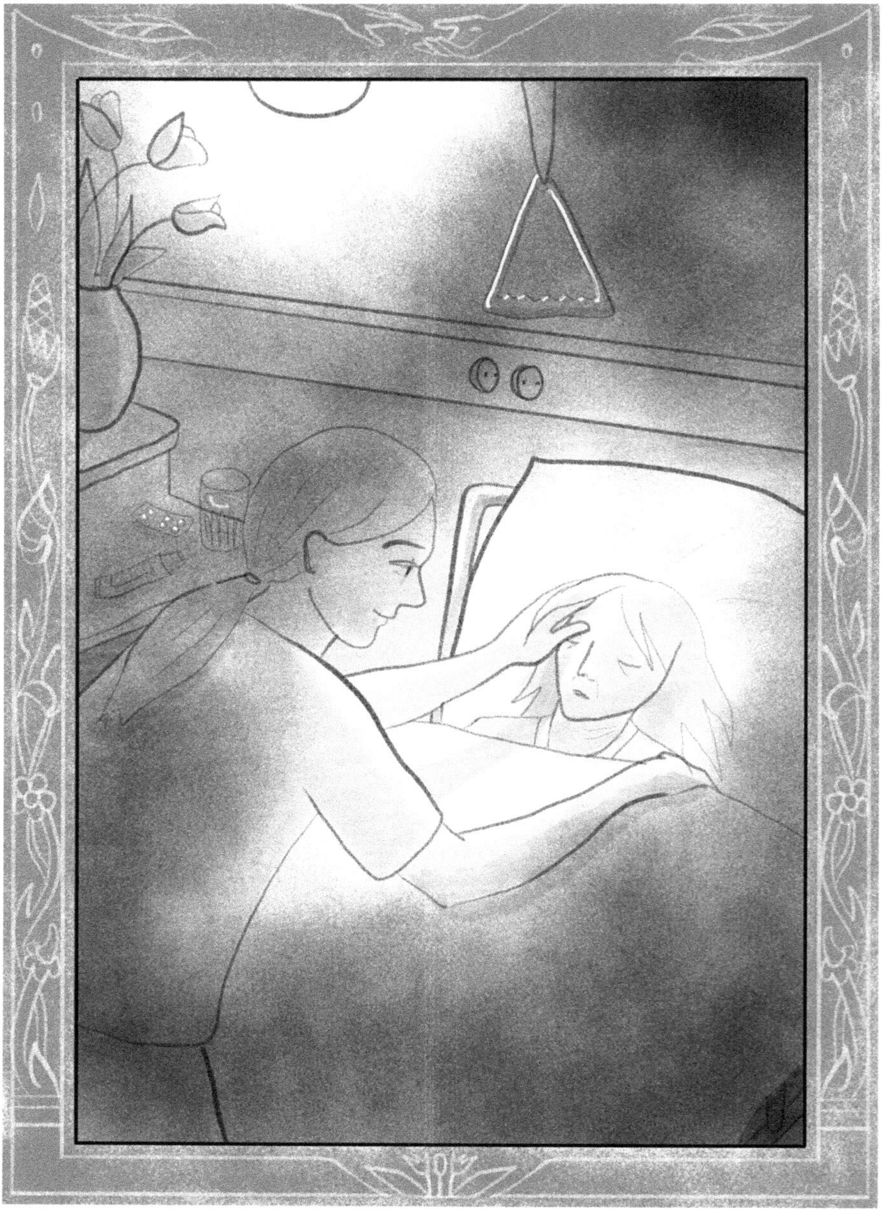

Figure 2.3 "Morality" (Illustration: Caroline Hamann).

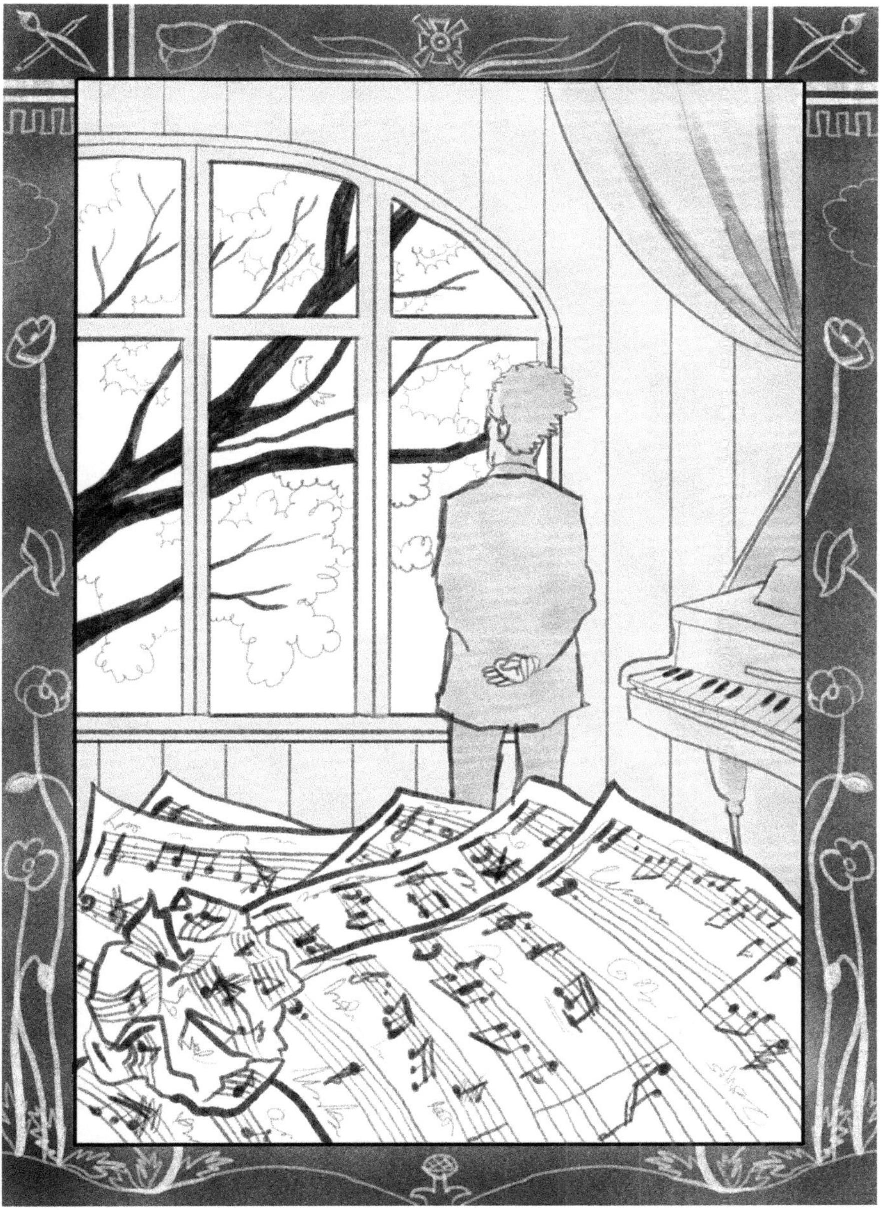

Figure 2.4 "Beauty" (Illustration: Caroline Hamann).

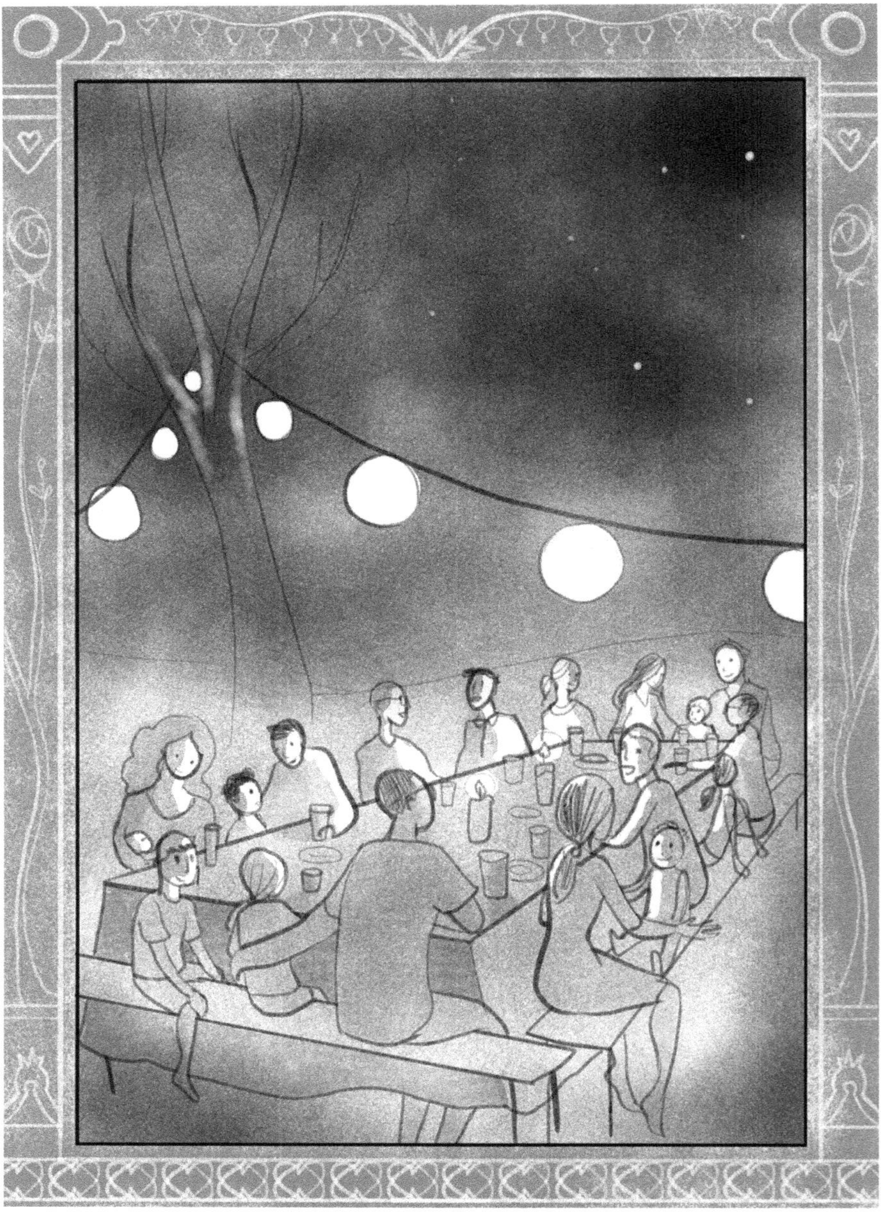

Figure 2.5 “Love” (Illustration: Caroline Hamann).

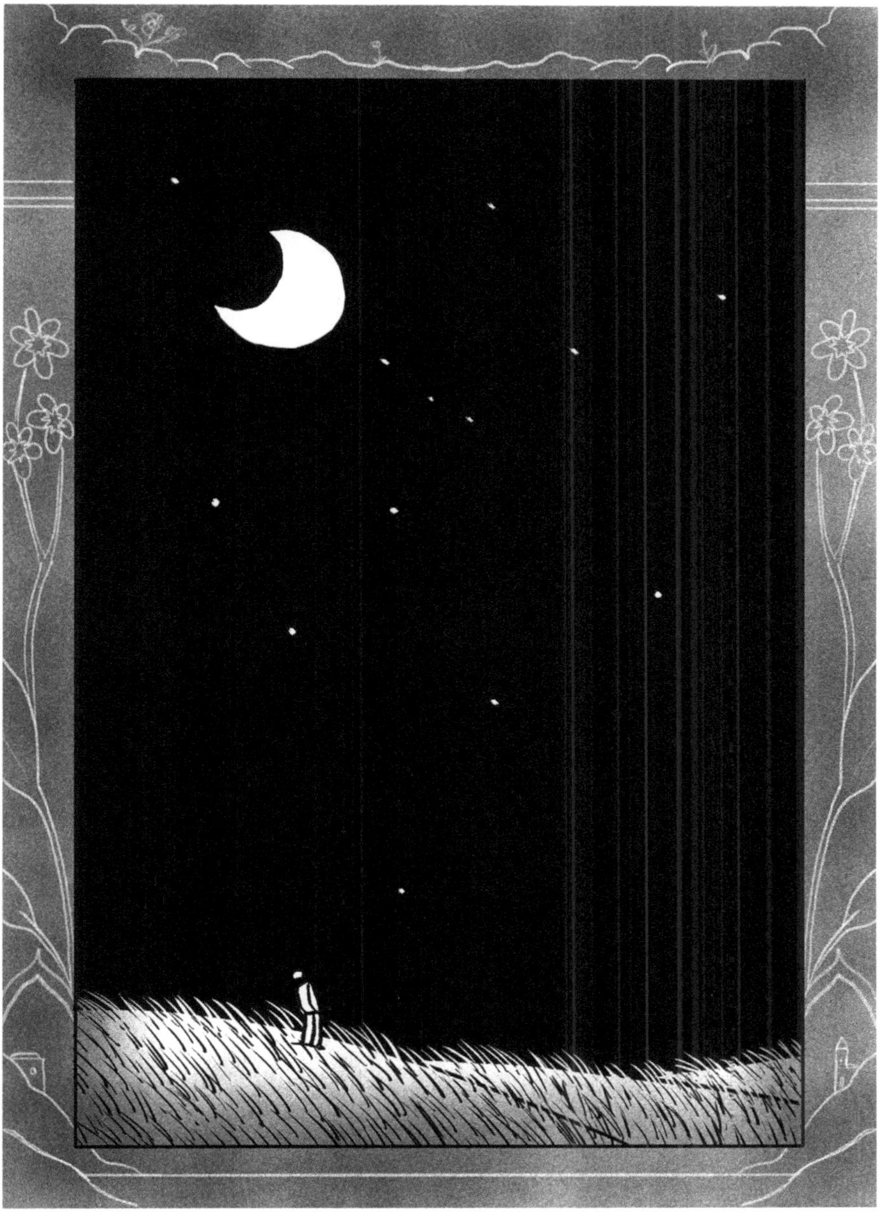

Figure 2.6 "Humility" (Illustration: Caroline Hamann).

about the purposes of life, since they will soon have to make life-shaping decisions about what to do after school. Yet, this consensus is, of course, flawed in two ways: First – despite all my efforts at participation – it is shaped by me, as the teacher, more than by the individual student. And second, it is biased in so far as the participants are concerned; we were all living in Germany, well-educated, on average fairly privileged, etc. Since I view the presented set of purposes of life as a result of this process,[5] and not so much as self-evident, these flaws also concern the set. Hence, it is unlikely that the set would have turned out exactly the same if someone other than me had led the process, and it is unlikely that it would be regarded as relevant as it seemed to us for people with a substantially different background. As a result, the set of purposes of life should be understood as *moderately epistemically ambitious*; the hope is that it seems relevant to many people who read it, but it does not claim to be self-evidently relevant for all people on earth, at all times.

Arguments for this three-fold position

Now, an answer to the question "What is the purpose of life?" has been given in three steps: First, a position about the form of the answer was presented, then the relation to each individual life was discussed, and finally, the content of the answer was briefly shown. Yet, the most important issue is still missing: Why should we hold this three-fold position? What are the arguments for it? In this section, I will present different arguments that – in my mind – suggest that this is a good philosophical position. They will be presented roughly in order of importance.

In my experience, the three-fold position is *productive*. Due to the fact that it is fairly concrete, it catches our interest, it gets constructive discussions going, it often makes one think seriously about one's own life. A big part of the reason why it does is the fact that it liberates the debate about the purpose of life from abstract issues that often inhibit intelligent debate about the topic: It deals with skepticism ("Of course life does not have a purpose!") not directly

5 Note that this is not the same as saying that the set resulted simply from asking people what they think about the purposes of life. Such an approach would certainly be an invalid inference from facts about peoples' opinions to the realm of the normative. That it is a consensus reached after long debate by reasonable people, though, is not such an invalid inference. To the contrary, in my opinion, such a method is one of the best ways to epistemically access the normative facts that exist for our lives.

but by presenting concrete options that are in some way well-known to us from our everyday experience; it is "down-to-earth" enough to evade the idea that thinking about the purpose of life is a highly abstract academical activity that does not make sense except to a few specialists; it does not allow the common "whatever floats your boat" attitude that in effect says that everyone can have anything they want as a purpose of life,[6] and thus this is not a matter worth talking about; and, again due to its concreteness, it prevents the reflexive negative answer that people often give when they say "we will never know the purpose of life, it's a mystery". Productivity or "being interesting", in my view, is one of the best arguments for any philosophical position. As William James puts it: "By its very essence, the reality of a thought is proportionate to the way it grasps us. Its intensity, its seriousness—its interest, in a word" (James 1878: 17).

There is a worry regarding realistically understood theories about the purposes of life, namely that any such a theory "opens the door to despotic requirements, externally imposed", as Robert Nozick says (Nozick 1993: 176). I believe this worry has two steps:

(A) If one holds an objective theory about purposes, this implies that one is entitled or even obliged to tell others how to lead their life.

(B) We should not hold or promote any theory that implies we should tell others how to live their lives, because it has a high potential to lead to morally bad actions (what Nozick calls "Despotism").

I agree with (B), but I believe that under the theory presented in this essay, (A) is not true. The two most important reasons are the following: First, the mosaic-view – since every person potentially has a very different, and partially radically self-created, way of giving importance to the different meanings of life, there is no one right way to live. This is especially true since this view includes the possibility of self-creation – thanks to this, even the possibility of someone else saying to me "I have studied your genes, your upbringing and your current circumstances, and thus I know what is best for you" is excluded. The second reason (A) is not implied by the position presented here are the moderate epistemic ambitions resulting from the method used; if another person does not seem to live according to any of the purposes of life set out here, it is more likely that they are following another really existing purpose – one that this theory simply has missed –, than that they are missing any purpose in their life.

---

6 Sometimes, this is called the "scope-problem" of desire-fulfillment theories of well-being", see Fletcher (2015).

There are some further reasons for this position to deny (A), which are less systematic but also important: Some of the shown purposes are such that it is very difficult or even impossible for another person to judge whether I live according to them, like humility or love. And, for each of the shown purposes, there are myriads of ways that they can be part of a human life: If, for example, I value "truth" very highly, I can become an academic. But I can also become an investigative journalist. Or I can focus on learning the truth about who I really am in some kind of deep introspective practice. And so on.

In a general sense, what was just said means that the position presented here is one in which objectively understood purposes of life are very much *compatible with individual human freedom.*

The position presented here can be classified as a kind of "objective list theory" of human well-being (see Crisp 2017, section 4.3). These theories are sometimes described as having (at least) two major problems, both of which the position presented here avoids. First, they can be seen as arbitrary (see Fletcher 2013), because we can always ask: "Why are exactly these items in the set?". This issue does not really arise for the present position, because it is only moderately epistemically ambitious: The question of why some other aspect is not on the list is something that should be reasonably discussed, and it is very well possible that as a result of that discussion, this aspect will end up being added to the list. But if it turned out that different discussions turn up very different sets of purposes, then the problem would return: It would seem arbitrary to choose one of these sets of purposes as somehow better than the others. At first, this problem seems very much to be real: Various lists proposed by various philosophers are never in complete congruence. John Finnis, for example, lists "Life", "Knowledge", "Play", "Aesthetic Experience", "Sociability (friendship)", "Practical reasonableness" and "'Religion'" (see Finnis 1980: 87 ff). Parfit's description of Frankfurt's "real view" lists "personal satisfaction, pleasure, glory, creativity, spiritual depth, and conformity with the requirements of morality" (Parfit 2011a: 55). James Griffin lists "Accomplishment", "the components of human existence", "Understanding", "Enjoyment" and "Deep personal relations" (see Griffin 1986: 67). And the position presented here lists "Happiness", "Truth", "Morality", "Beauty", "Love" and "Humility". At first glance, the four lists seem very different: Why not include "spiritual depth" in my list? Why not include "Morality" in Finnis' list? Upon deeper reflection, though, these different lists actually prove the opposite: In my list, "Humility" is conceived in a spiritual way (Andrae 2018: 140) – hence, in a way, it shares this aspect with the other lists. And for Finnis, an important aspect of "practical reasonableness" is acting in "accordance with one's conscience" (Finnis 1980: 125). In many such ways, I claim, it actually turns out that the *different lists express many of the same basic ideas* – this is especially striking if, as was the case for the position presented here, they were developed without explicit knowledge of the other lists.

The second major problem that objective list theories are usually considered to have is that under them it is (theoretically) possible to live a good life that one does not oneself have any positive reaction to (see Rice 2013): If I despise art but somehow end up producing it at a really high level, then, this worry claims, according to an objective list theory, I do lead a very good life. This seems counter-intuitive. However, the mosaic nature differentiates the position presented here from ones that are susceptible to this criticism because this entails that *although the purposes of life are realistically understood and therefore independent of the individual human and their mental states, which of them apply to which human is not.* The present position even claims that there always is some positivity in my mental states, known to me or not, that can tell me which purposes of life are really for me – thus directly contradicting this objection.

The final argument I will present is taken from our everyday experience: The present position has the advantage of allowing an individual *some flexibility when it comes to the purposes of life.* If circumstances make it difficult or even impossible to follow one of my central purposes, according to the position presented here, I can – via self-creation – over time change myself into a person for whom other, more attainable purposes take center stage. This flexibility is something that each of us needs in our personal lives from time to time, and thus it is good if a theoretical position leaves room for it. To give two examples: If love is one of my central purposes of life, but then my partner and my friends leave me, I can use the free time to really get into art and eventually turn myself into a person for whom beauty is the main purpose of life. Or, if truth is one of the things that give my life purpose, but due to the drying up of research funds I lose my job at the university, I can learn to appreciate the time spent with my family and friends more and thus become someone who focusses very much on love as a purpose of life.

Outlook

Let me end by saying what the position presented in this essay does *not* do: It does not answer the question "Why are the purposes presented such as they are?" If this question is understood as looking for an underlying reason that somehow grounds the goodness of the purposes presented in a more basic purpose or value, then it is misguided; because these purposes are conceived as ends in themselves that make other things good, the question "but why are they good?" does not make sense anymore. However, if the question is understood as an attempt to systematize the theory a bit better, to understand what the different purposes might have in common, then it certainly is interesting – because obviously the different purposes are not completely unrelated, but in some ways seem quite connected: Love usually makes me happy, Truth is often considered beautiful or humbling, Morality can be understood as the duty to enable others to follow the different purposes of their lives, and so on. This indicates that an attempt to understand the things many or even all the different purposes have in common might prove fruitful and illuminating. Although I will not spell this out in detail, it seems to me that one interesting aspect that many of the purposes presented here have in common is some kind of transcendence of the human ego: Learning a truth means becoming part of something that is beyond the human person, art is often described in terms of artists being merely facilitators of some force other than themselves, in Morality we take the perspective of others and think "what would it be like if I was in their place", in Love we often say that someone else is more important to us than even ourselves, and in Humility we attempt not to consider ourselves too important.

Bibliography

Andrae B (2018) Die Sinne des Lebens. München: Philosophia Verlag.

Brüntrup G (2020) Was uns antreibt (online), Die Neue Vernunft Magazin (Zitierdatum 04.08.20), abrufbar unter https://die-neue-vernunft.de/magazin-interview-mit-bruntrup/.

Callard A (2018) Aspiration. Oxford: Oxford University Press (cited from the 2019 paperback edition).

Crisp R (2017) Well-Being. The Stanford Encyclopedia of Philosophy (Fall 2017 Edition), Edward N. Zalta (ed.), URL = https://plato.stanford.edu/archives/fall2017/entries/well-being/.

Finnis J (1980) Natural Law & Natural Rights. Oxford: Oxford University Press (cited from the second edition in paperback 2011).

Frankl E (1959) Man's search for meaning. Boston: Beacon Press. (Cited from the 2006 Edition, translated by Ilse Lasch).

Fletcher G (2013) A Fresh Start for the Objective-List Theory of Well-Being. Cambridge: Cambridge University Press, Utilitas Vol. 25, No. 2

Fletcher G (2015) Objective List Theories. In: The Routledge Handbook of Philosophy of Well-Being. Abingdon: Routledge.

Griffin D R (2001) Reenchantment without Supernaturalism. New York: Cornell University Press.

Griffin J (1986) Well-Being. Oxford: Oxford University Press.

James W (1878) Remarks on Spencer's Definition of Mind as Correspondence. The Journal of Speculative Philosophy, vol. 12, no. 1, Jan. 1878, pp. 1–18.

Mintz-Woo K (2018) On Parfit's Ontology, Canadian Journal of Philosophy, 48:5, 707–725.
Nozick R (1993) The Nature of Rationality. Princeton: Princeton University Press.
Parfit D (2011a) On What Matters, Volume 1. Oxford: Oxford University Press (cited from the 2013 paperback edition).
Parfit D (2011b) On What Matters, Volume 2. : Oxford: Oxford University Press (cited from the 2013 paperback edition).
Rice C M (2013) Defending the Objective List Theory of Well-Being. Ratio, 26: 196–211.
Russell B (1903) A Free Man's Worship, cited from "Betrand Russell: Mysticism and Logic and other essays", London: George Allen & Unwin.
Whitehead A N (1938) Modes of Thought. New York: The Free Press, Cited from the 1968 Free Press edition.
Whitehead A N (1929) Process and Reality. New York: The Free Press, Cited from the 1979 Free Press edition.

Eckhard Frick

Über den Sinn des Lebens reden

Talking about the Meaning of Life

Zusammenfassung: Niklas Luhmann kritisiert die Definition des Menschen durch ein Bedürfnis, seinem Leben einen Sinn zu geben, ein Bedürfnis, das von Religion und Spiritualität erfüllt wird. Das Religionssystem bezieht sich auf die der Differenz zwischen immanent (markiert, beobachtbar, positiv) und transzendent (unmarkiert, unbeobachtbar, negativ) zu Grunde liegende Einheit. Das Unmarkierte („Schatten" nach C.G. Jung) wird für gewöhnlich aus der aktiven Sinngebung ausgeschlossen, weil fälschlicherweise angenommen wird, dass Sinn immer Wohlbefinden hervorrufen sollte. Christlicher Glaube widersteht der Versuchung der aktiven Sinnerzeugung in der Auseinandersetzung mit der scheinbaren Absurdität von Leiden und Sterben.

Schlüsselwörter: Luhmann, C.G. Jung, Sinngebung, Spiritual Care, Religion

Abstract: Niklas Luhmann criticises the definition of the human being by reference to a need to give one's life meaning, a need responded to by religion and spirituality. The religious system refers to the unity of the difference between immanent (marked, observable, positive) and transcendent (unmarked, unobservable, negative). The unmarked ("shadow" according to C.G. Jung) is commonly excluded from active meaning-making, due to the bias that meaning should always provide well-being. Christian faith resists the temptation of meaning-making when facing the apparent absurdity of suffering and dying.

Keywords: Luhmann, C.G. Jung, meaning-making, spiritual care, religion

Wir wollen über die Sinnfrage nachdenken, insbesondere über die Instrumentalisierung der Sinnfrage in Medizin und Psychotherapie. Sinn gehört zu den meliorativen Begriffen, ist normativ aufgeladen: Sinn soll / muss gefunden oder therapeutisch hergestellt werden. Die Bipolarität von Sinn, der „dunkle Sinn" (Vogel 2021) wird von vornherein aus dem Diskurs ausgeschlossen. Abwesenheit von Sinn gilt als *spiritual distress*, als behandlungsbedürftiges Symptom. Besonders normativ ist die Erfindung des Sterbenden: Der Sterbende soll akzeptieren, Sinn finden, generativ sein, dann darf er mit dem Sterben aufhören und endlich tot sein (Saake et al. 2019). Wenigstens am Schluss muss der Mensch Sinn

https://doi.org/10.1515/9783110787153-003

finden, wenigstens am Schluss soll er doch akzeptieren, soll er doch generativ sein, soll er doch sich versöhnen und dann darf er abtreten.

Sinn als Differenzbegriff

Luhmann versteht unter einem System dessen Differenz gegenüber der Umwelt eben dieses Systems. Oder: Jede Grenzziehung oder Markierung ergibt eine Differenz zwischen dem markierten Innenbereich des Systems und dem sie umgebenden *unmarked space*. Oder: Sinn ist Formgebung, Differenz von Medium und Form. Systeme funktionieren jeweils durch die binäre Codierung zwischen markiert und unmarkiert, z. B. krank vs. gesund (Luhmann 1990); recht vs. unrecht (Recht) oder immanent vs. transzendent (Religionssystem).

Man kann sagen, dass jede Grenzziehung oder jede Markierung einen unmarkierten Bereich „braucht"; jeder *marked space* braucht einen *unmarked space* (Spencer-Brown 1971) oder aber: Sinn ist Formgebung, Differenz zwischen einem unsichtbaren Medium und einer sichtbaren Form oder Gestalt (Luhmann 2002/2017: 226). Eine mögliche Sinn-Definition (*de-finitio* heißt: Bestimmung einer *finis:* Grenze, Ende, Ziel von etwas) besteht darin, archetypische Sinn-Situationen abzubilden und folglich einzurahmen, also gegen das Nicht-Abgebildete abzugrenzen (Andrae 2018). Was jedoch ist außerhalb des Rahmens? Worin besteht die Differenz zwischen den Bildern? Wenn wir diese situative Sinn-Definition anwenden, dann sind wir bezüglich der Sinne des Lebens „im Bilde", aber eben nur, weil es auch das Außerhalb des Bildes und jenseits der gewählten Form das Medium gibt.

Dass Sinn Differenz ist und nicht etwas Substanzielles oder Phänomenales, bringt Luhmann mit dem Horizont der Verweisung auf andere Möglichkeiten, mit der Appräsentation anderer Möglichkeiten (Husserl) in Verbindung:

> Aber Sinn ist nicht nur dieses Verweisen auf andere Möglichkeiten, sondern auch die Lokalisierung dieser Verweisung in allem, was wir uns konkret als Gegenstand unserer Aktualität, unseres aktuellen Erlebens vorstellen. [...] Alle Items, die operativ aktualisiert werden, leben und haben Sinn nur, weil sie in einem Horizont anderer Möglichkeiten platziert sind (Luhmann 2002/2017: 231).

Religion und Spiritualität: Zwischen Sinn-Realismus und Sinn-Despotismus

„Ob mein Leben sinnvoll ist, entscheidet die Welt und nicht ich als Subjekt" (Benjamin Andrae in diesem Band). Luhmann beschreibt soziale Systeme als Kommunikationssysteme, die Sinn produzieren, und zwar über die Köpfe der Subjekte hinweg. Diese Betrachtungsweise ist ungewohnt, gehen wir doch meist davon aus, dass Sinn psychische Systeme betrifft, Bewusstseins-Systeme, die Sinn erleben. Inwiefern ist mit der systemischen Sinnproduktion ein Sinn-Despotismus verknüpft, wird dem Subjekt als Sinn aufoktroyiert, was der gesellschaftliche Konsens für sinnvoll hält? Geben wir z. B. den Sterbenden einen Sinnauftrag, wir, die wir zwar auch Sterbende sind, aber nach unserer Vermutung noch weiter vom Tod entfernt als die von uns konstruierten „Sterbenden" (Saake et al. 2019)?

Einer der großen Sinnagenten unserer Gesellschaft ist das Religionssystem, das nach dem binären Code immanent vs. transzendent funktioniert. Nun beobachtet Luhmann mit Spencer Brown, dass die Differenz zwischen markiertem und unmarkiertem Bereich innerhalb des markierten Bereichs wiederkehrt (Reentry). Auf die Religion bezogen: Kirchen, Moscheen und Synagogen sind vollkommen weltliche, immanente Einrichtungen. Wir begegnen in diesen Gebäuden nicht der Transzendenz, die ja außerhalb unseres markierten, immanenten Bereichs liegt. Wir überschreiten in keinem religiösen Gebäude die Grenze zum unmarkierten Bereich. Und doch werden wir auf Schritt und Tritt auf die Leitdifferenz hingewiesen (Frick 2019).

Luhmann weist immer wieder auf die spezifische Funktion der Religion bezüglich der Differenz zwischen markiertem und unmarkiertem Bereich hin. Diese Differenz bringt Sinn hervor:

> Wie immer die Grenze zwischen marked und unmarked gezogen wird: als Religion kann uns nur eine Sinngebung gelten, die genau darin ihr Problem sieht. Das heißt vor allem: dass jeder Formgebrauch Religion involviert, da jeder Formgebrauch einen unmarked state erzeugt.
> (Ohne Markierung gäbe es selbstverständlich auch nichts „Unmarkiertes"; die Welt muss immer zuerst durch die Unterscheidung markiert/unmarkiert in einen imaginären Raum transformiert werden.) Aber dennoch hat Religion bei universaler Sinnzuständigkeit eine spezifische Unterscheidung im Auge, eben die von marked/unmarked (beobachtbar/unbeobachtbar). Doch wie kann dies als eine Unterscheidung bezeichnet, als eine Form markiert werden, wenn sich die andere Seite, die Außenseite der Unterscheidung, der Markierung entzieht und genau dies die Bedingung der Markierung selbst ist?
> (Luhmann 2002: 53).

Sinn als nicht-negierbare Kategorie

Die „universale Sinnzuständigkeit“ der Religion betrifft auch Lebens- und gesellschaftliche Funktionsbereiche, die auf den ersten Blick nicht „religiös“ genannt werden. Die Universalisierung der Sinn-Anforderung, die normative Aufladung von Sinn als eines meliorativen, schattenlosen Begriffs zeigt Luhmann zufolge eine „Sinnlosigkeitsklage“, aber auch den Legitimationsdruck von Einzelpersonen und Organisationen, Sinn vorhalten und generieren zu müssen, z. B. in Leitbildern, Internet-Auftritten, Corporate Identity und Organisationskultur (Luhmann 2002/2017: 246). Sinn als nicht-negierbare Kategorie: Die Sinnlosigkeitsklage ist das Korrelat eines gesellschaftlichen Sinn-Oktrois, das sich in der positiven Konnotierung, in der Meliorisierung des Sinnbegriffs äußert. Je mehr Rechenschaft wir geben müssen, je mehr wir unter Legitimationsdruck geraten, je mehr wir sagen müssen, worin der eigentliche Sinn besteht, sei es unseres eigenen Lebens, sei es einer Institution, eines Teils einer Organisation oder des gesellschaftlichen Lebens insgesamt, desto mehr wird die Differenz von sinnvoll/sinnlos oktroyiert.

Das Nichtmarkierte, das Ausgeschlossene können wir mit Jung den Schatten nennen, die Summe der ungelebten Möglichkeiten, den Dinosaurierschwanz des kultivierten Menschen (siehe Jung GW 11: § 140 und Vogel in diesem Band). „Schatten“ ist für Jung keineswegs nur das moralisch Abgewertete und deshalb auf missliebige Mitmenschen Projizierte, sondern auch das Nicht-Gelebte, um das wir möglicherweise andere beneiden oder weshalb wir andere kritisieren. Auch dies ist eine Differenzerfahrung, in diesem Fall nicht zwischen Markiert und Unmarkiert oder Form und Hintergrund, sondern zwischen dem Individuum und seiner Welt, d. h. den anderen. Solange der Schatten nicht angenommen ist, wird er projiziert, im Außen gesucht, dort kritisiert, behandelt und bekämpft. Auch dadurch entsteht Sinn, können wir in Analogie zu Luhmann sagen, indem wir unsere helle Seite gegenüber dem nicht angenommenen und projizierten Schatten abgrenzen. Der Schatten ist für Jung das ungelebte Leben. Das funktionelle Äquivalent dessen, was Luhmann das Nichtmarkierte nennt, ist in Jungs archetypischer Psychologie der Schatten, das Nicht-Gewählte, das Ungeliebte, das Projizierte, das Delegierte, alles, was ich nicht sein will und doch bin.

Jung vergleicht die Lebenskurve mit der Parabel, die ein Wurfgeschoss beschreibt: der Scheitelpunkt ist der Lebensmittag, danach geht es bergab, wenn auch zunächst unmerklich oder verleugnet. Die Normativität des Sinnbegriffs hat hier eine Wurzel: wir konstruieren Sinn nach einem Aufstiegsschema und versuchen, die Sinnlosigkeiten unseres Lebens als Wachstum und Aufstieg umzudeuten, gewissermaßen als Jungbrunnen, aus dem neuer Sinn fließt:

> Dem Aufstieg des Lebens billigen wir Ziel und Sinn zu, warum nicht dem Abstieg? Die Geburt des Menschen ist bedeutungsschwanger, warum nicht der Tod? Der junge Mensch wird zwanzig und mehr Jahre auf die völlige Entfaltung seiner Einzelexistenz vorbereitet, warum soll er sich nicht zwanzig und mehr Jahre auf sein Ende vorbereiten? Allerdings – mit dem Höhepunkt hat man es sichtlich erreicht, man ist's und man hat's. Was ist aber mit dem Tod erreicht? (GW 8: § 803).

Sinn in der Krankheit: Ergebung oder Protest?

Nicht erst am Lebensende, sondern allgemein im Umgang mit Krankheit wird Spiritual Care mit der Sinnfrage oder *meaning making* (Hvidt 2012; Timmins & Caldeira 2019) verknüpft. Luhmann kritisiert die (anthropologische) Rede vom „Menschen", der durch sein Bedürfnis nach Sinn definiert wird. Sinnsuche, Wunsch nach der Gewissheit eines sinnvollen Lebens werden ihm ebenso unterstellt wie die Negierung von Sinnleere und Sinnlosigkeit. Religion ist als Einzelsystem und zugleich universalisiert in allen Funktionssystemen das gesellschaftliche „Angebot, das auf diesen Sinnbedarf reagiert" (Luhmann 2002: 340) oder im Sinne des psycho-spirituellen Sinnmarktes diesen Sinnbedarf erzeugt. Die Säkularisierungstendenzen westlicher Gesellschaften ändern an dieser grundsätzlichen soziologischen Struktur nichts. Vielmehr ist die Anthropologie des sinnbedürftigen und sinnverpflichteten Menschen die säkularisierte Gestalt des Religionssystems. Indem Luhmann eine anthropologische, möglicherweise essentialistische Zugangsweise zur Sinnproblematik kritisiert und ironisiert, deckt er die durch gesellschaftliche Normierung gleichzeitig blockierte und verdeckte Individualisierung des „Meaning-making" auf. Der Mensch wird individualisiert, abstrahiert von den Maschinerien gesellschaftlicher Sinnkonstruktion gesehen. Damit in eins geht eine Selbstbeschreibung des Systems Religion, welches sich in Differenz zur säkularisierten Umwelt sieht. Sinnbedarf ist Ausdruck dieser Säkularisierung, tritt an die Stelle früherer Charakterisierungen wie zum Beispiel Sündigkeit und Vergebungsbedürfnis:

> Die alte Sorge um Heil und Erlösung kann fast bruchlos entdogmatisiert und in die neu konzipierte Sorge um Sinn überführt werden. Dabei ist ‚der Mensch' eine Fiktion, der keine Realität entspricht. Die ungeheure Vielfalt individueller Erlebniswelten aller Zeiten wird systematisch verkannt, entsprechende Informationen werden systematisch unterdrückt oder ‚vergessen'. Der ‚dem Menschen' unterstellte Sinnbedarf ist schon die Deutung, auf die die Religion eine Antwort zu geben hofft. Die Problemlösung liegt im Formenschatz der Religion und in der Rede von ‚Heil' und ‚Erlösung' bereits vor, nur das Problem wird hinzuerfunden (Luhmann 2002: 340).

Die Befriedigung eines Sinnbedürfnisses als säkularisierte Religion ist auch in theologischer Hinsicht kritisch zu sehen. Deshalb kritisiert Josuttis logotherapeutische Versuche einer Sinnzuschreibung in Krankheit und Leid als Werkgerechtigkeit: Das Leiden werde hier als „die höchste und letzte Möglichkeit des Menschen" missverstanden, „das eigene Leben in den Griff zu bekommen" und „sinnloses Geschehen in Sinn zu verwandeln". Weil aber für den Glauben der Sinn des menschlichen Lebens Gott selber ist und nicht das Resultat eigener Anstrengungen (theologisch: „Werke"), sei der Glaube nicht Kraft zur Sinndeutung, sondern „Kraft zum Verzicht auf Sinndeutung in religiöser Hinsicht" (Josuttis 1974: 130). Wenn Spiritual Care vorwiegend oder sogar ausschließlich als sinnzentriertes „Meaning making" verstanden wird, droht die Gefahr von säkularisierter Werkgerechtigkeit und Selbsterlösung. Soziologisch gesprochen, soll mit dem normativen Sinn-Oktroi am Souveränitätsparadigma der Moderne festgehalten werden. Der individuelle und kollektive Konflikt zwischen Kontrollierenwollen auf der einen und In-Resonanz-Gehen mit dem Unverfügbaren auf der anderen Seite wird dadurch einseitig in Richtung der Machbarkeit um jeden Preis (pseudo-)gelöst. Im Sinne einer „spirituellen Abhängigkeitserklärung" (Rosa 2019) wird jedoch zunehmend die Notwendigkeit des einseitigen Souveränitätsparadigmas und des Übergangs in ein „mediopassives Weltverhältnis, das ebenso gut ein medioaktives genannt werden kann" (Rosa 2019), deutlich. Dies heißt (erkenntnistheoretisch) in der Wahrnehmung und (therapeutisch-praktisch) in der Interventionsplanung: Sinnfremdes ist nicht sinnhaft, kann nicht in Sinn transformiert werden (s. Lampersberger in diesem Band). Sinn entsteht nicht durch Psychologisierung oder Spiritualisierung von Leid, also durch äußere Zuschreibung, etwa durch Appelle wie: „Krankheit als Chance", „Sie müssen jetzt loslassen!", „Das Leben geht weiter". Vielmehr geschieht existenzielle Transformation von Sinnlosigkeit in Sinn nur, wo und wann sie möglich ist und nur durch den leidenden Menschen selbst. Insofern entlastet die Befreiung vom Sinn-Oktroi den kranken Menschen vom inneren, in der persönlichen Geschichte angelegten, und vom äußeren, durch gesellschaftliche Normierung entstehenden Zwang:

> Die Krankheit an sich hat keinerlei Sinn. Jeder Versuch, ihr einen Sinn zuzuschreiben, will ihr den Schrecken nehmen, der über die körperlichen Schmerzen hinausreicht, den Schrecken der Sinnlosigkeit. Die Sinndeutung der Krankheit ist deshalb nicht nur, psychologisch gesehen, eine Flucht vor der Härte einer aussichtslosen Realität, sie ist darüber hinaus, in den Kategorien der Rechtfertigungslehre gesprochen, das Werk der Selbsterlösung aus der Sinnlosigkeit (Josuttis 1974: 129).

Wenn wir Sinn mit Luhmann als eine kommunikative Eigenschaft gesellschaftlicher Systeme und nicht als Leistung eines Subjekts auffassen, so kann uns dies demütig machen. Zweifellos kommen beim Sinnerleben und „meaning making" auch psychische Systeme ins Spiel. Doch lässt sich von Luhmann lernen, wie die gesellschaftlichen Systeme in ihren Leitunterscheidungen im Umgang mit den Differenzen ständig Sinn produzieren und damit auch eine gewisse Macht ausüben. Sinn ist ein meliorativer, normativ aufgeladener Begriff, der deshalb mit so viel Leuchtkraft ausgestattet wird, weil er sich gegen die Dunkelheit des unmarked space abhebt. Weil wir so einen hellen Sinn konstruieren müssen, gibt es auch diesen anderen Bereich, diesen Schatten des Sinnfremden, des Schattens, der bei dieser Debatte nicht vergessen werden darf. Insbesondere das Religionssystem „macht Sinn", aber auch Spiritual Care in der Medizin. Die Doppeldeutigkeit dieses Amerikanismus im Deutschen weist auf die Tendenz hin, dass meaning making für gesellschaftliche Produktion von Sinn steht und damit für den Sinn-Despotismus. Das sinnsuchende Subjekt wieder in seine Rechte einzusetzen, muss freilich nicht heißen, in das von Josuttis kritisierte Extrem der Selbsterlösung aus Sinnlosigkeit zu verfallen. Eine realitätsnahe, geerdete Mystik setzt sich mit dem „grausamen Un-Sinn des Lebens" auseinander, wovon in einem unveröffentlichten Brief Karl Rahners an Luise Rinser (30.1.65, 17.15 abends, p.M. Bruno Lautenschlager) die Rede ist:

> Die wahre Mystik ersetzt und verdrängt das diesseitige Leben nicht, sondern gibt ihm eine Tiefe und Erlöstheit, lässt es aber bestehen. Denn Gott ist nicht ein Stück der Welt. Und wenn einer einsam ist, müde und verloren, dann ist es falsch zu sagen: bete (und so weiter). Denn das tut er ja (unter Umständen). Aber die Welt (zu der auch der Nächste und der Fernste gehören) muss doch getan und erlitten werden. Krebs, Alter, Einsamkeit. Der wahre Gott fungiert nicht als Analgetikum dafür. Nur als Erlösung der getanen und erlittenen Welt. Das landläufige Christentum erniedrigt Gott oft zu diesem „Lückenbüßer" (um mit Robinson zu sprechen) und macht ihn so unglaubwürdig. In Wirklichkeit umfasst er den grausamen Un-Sinn des Lebens, hebt diesen aber nicht auf. Das Kreuz Christi ist ja nicht die erfahrene, sondern geglaubte Überwindung des Todes dieser Welt in allen seinen Gestalten. „Es wird schon besser"; dieses Wort ist falsch. Es wird immer schlechter, bis man stirbt. Aber dieser Schmerz des Todes, der sich hinzieht, setzt sich als seine Möglichkeit voraus den Protest, das Anders Habenwollen, den wütenden Hunger nach Nähe, Leben, Heiterkeit. Sonst wäre er ja gar nicht möglich. Das Tote kann nicht sterben. Aber die Einsicht in diese Dialektik hebt den Schmerz nicht auf. Die Gottverlassenheit Christi war nicht gelindert durch sein Wissen, dass er allzeit beim Vater ist und in seine Hände fällt. Das bilden sich nur harmlose Aszeten und Spirituäle ein, bis – auch sie ans Sterben kommen (Meist haben sie dann keine Möglichkeit mehr, ihre bisher verdrängte Erfahrung kund zu machen). Wodurch unterscheidet sich also das Sterben des rechten und des linken Schächers? Nicht durch die Qual des Sterbens. Der Unterschied ist empirisch nicht mehr recht nachweisbar (dort, wo das Letzte geschieht) und eigentlich ist es nur Gott bekannt. Die Christen sollten mehr Mut haben, zu verzweifeln. Dann erst begännen sie recht zu glauben.

Diskussion

Lässt sich Sinn als Differenz (markiert vs. unmarkiert; Form vs. Medium) auch in umgekehrter Richtung verstehen?

Wie man Luhmanns *binary codes* versteht, hat auch etwas mit Konvention zu tun. Bezüglich der Medizin ist Luhmanns Differenzierung besonders erstaunlich: Markiert ist das Kranke, Unmarkiert das Gesunde, nicht umgekehrt:

> Wenn es ein Code sein soll, muß ein Positivwert und ein Negativwert nachweisbar sein, so daß die Operationen durch eine Asymmetrie strukturiert werden. Der Positivwert vermittelt die Anschlußfähigkeit der Operationen des Systems, der Negativwert vermittelt die Kontingenzreflexion, also die Vorstellung, es könnte auch anders sein. Im Anwendungsbereich des Systems der Krankenbehandlung kann dies nur heißen: der positive Wert ist die Krankheit, der negative Wert die Gesundheit. Nur Krankheiten sind für den Arzt instruktiv, nur mit Krankheiten kann er etwas anfangen. Die Gesundheit gibt nichts zu tun, sie reflektiert allenfalls das, was fehlt, wenn jemand krank ist. Entsprechend gibt es viele Krankheiten und nur eine Gesundheit. Die Krankheitsterminologien wachsen mit der Medizin, und der Begriff der Gesundheit wird zugleich problematisch und inhaltsleer. Gesunde sind, medizinisch gesehen, noch nicht oder nicht mehr krank oder sie leiden an noch unentdeckten Krankheiten. Wenn Ärzte Gesundheit differenziert überprüfen müssen – etwa bei Einberufung in den Militärdienst oder unter dem Gesichtspunkt der „Tropentauglichkeit", dann geschieht das typisch im Hinblick auf die Anforderungen anderer Funktionssysteme und nicht zu Heilzwecken (Luhmann 1990: 179).

Hinsichtlich der Kodierung krank vs. gesund spricht Luhmann selbst von einer „Absonderlichkeit", von einer „perversen Vertauschung der Werte", die damit zusammenhänge, dass in der Medizin der Negativwert „Gesundheit" keiner Reflexion bedürfe und die Medizin „keine auf ihre Funktion bezogene Reflexionstheorie ausgebildet" habe, im Unterschied zu den Reflexionswerten Transzendenz in der Theologie und Unwahrheit in der Erkenntnistheorie der Wissenschaft (180). Weil die Teleologie der Medizin (Beseitigung oder wenigstens Linderung von Krankheit) unwidersprochen ist und sich, vor allem bei *akutem* Auftreten gebieterisch in den Vordergrund schiebt, ist der Negativwert des medizinischen Codes (die Gesundheit) merkwürdig unreflektiert, was zur Autonomie des Gesundheitssystems und zur medizinischen Sinnkonstruktion beiträgt. Vor allem da, wo die Medizin „nichts mehr machen kann", wird die Sinnfrage virulent. Vorher, z. B. im Umgang mit einer sinnfremden Pandemie, ist technische Rationalität gefragt.

Auch unabhängig davon, ob die Sinnfrage gestellt wird, entsteht Sinn durch die Differenz, durch das Auswählen des Markierten in Abhebung vom schattenhaften Unmarkierten. Sinn entsteht demnach schon durch die Diagnose, z. B.

indem ich Infizierte von Nicht-Infizierten unterscheide und dann nach einer nachvollziehbaren Rationale vorgehe. Die Infektion durch ein Virus ist ebenso sinnfremd wie ein Tumor oder eine genetisch verursachte Erkrankung, erst die Differenz „schafft" Sinn.

Ist die Deutung des Nichtmarkierten als Schatten zu kategorial?

In der Tat verlangen Luhmanns Kodierungen ein binäres Entweder-Oder, während die Metapher des Schattens oder der Dunkelheit auch Übergänge, *Schattierungen* kennt. Im konventionellen Kunstbetrieb ist beispielsweise ein Gemälde mit seinem Rahmen eindeutig von der Wand / der Tapete abgegrenzt, auf der es hängt. Man kann mit dieser kategorialen Disjunktion aber auch spielen: Installationskunst oder Performance schafft erst einmal Unsicherheit darüber, ob und wann ich beim Eintreten in einen Raum Kunst vorfinde. Vielleicht befinde ich mich plötzlich im Vorraum einer Toilette. Die Toilette selbst kann künstlerische Elemente umfassen, etwa dadurch, dass mir vorgespiegelt wird, in die Toilette eines anderen Geschlechts eingetreten zu sein.

Das Spielen mit den Grenzen kann sich im Theater durch die bewegliche Bühne inszenieren, welche die Zuschauer plötzlich auf der Bühne sitzen lassen, während die Schauspieler von hinten rufen. Das Verschieben der Grenze bestätigt die Leitdifferenz.

Gibt es ein vorbildliches, würdevolles, inspirierendes Sterben?

Wir müssen mit der Spannung zwischen der Autonomie sterbender Menschen und dem Despotismus der Gesellschaft leben, der sich nicht zuletzt in der Ökonomisierung von Palliative Care zeigt, berechnet in standardisierten Verweildauern, innerhalb derer gestorben werden muss (jedenfalls im statistischen Mittel), oder aber die Entlassung / Verlegung zu erfolgen hat). Der Mittelwert ist hier wie in der übrigen Medizin ein Steuerungselement. Dies steht in einer Spannung zur Geschichte der Palliativ- und Hospizbewegung, die aus einem bürgerschaftlichen Engagement entsteht und nun unverhofft sowohl in medizinische als auch in wirtschaftliche Systemzwänge eingepasst wird. Und dies zeigt sich auch auf der Seite der betroffenen Sterbenden: Geben wir ihnen so viel Freiheitsraum, wie angesichts begrenzter Lebenszeit möglich?

Führt die Sinnsuche zu größerer oder geringerer Freiheit des Subjektes?

Durch die normative Aufladung des Sinnbegriffs ist die Sinnsuche anfällig für mehr oder minder bewusste Machtausübung, für Ideologisierung und Ökonomisierung. Deshalb werden in diesem Beitrag soziologische, philosophische und theologische Einwände gegen systemische Sinnproduktionen und deren normative Überhöhung formuliert.

Wenn dem Subjekt Sinnsuche, „meaning making", Sinngefühl als Normen aufgebürdet werden, entsteht nicht nur eine terminologische Verkürzung des Sinn-Konzeptes, sondern auch ein gegen die Individuation gerichteter Machtmissbrauch. Erst wenn anerkannt wird, dass „Sinn" die engen Grenzen des Subjekts transzendiert (Stein 2022) und dunkle, vordergründig „sinnlose" Aspekte umfasst (Vogel 2022), ist der Weg zum Sinn wieder frei.

Am Ende lässt sich sagen, dass die Konstruktion von Sinn eine ambivalente Sache ist: Sie kann ein System dadurch „schmieren", dass die Subjekte den kollektiven Sinnvorgaben angepasst werden, und sei es dadurch, dass ihre Freiheit auf die Wahlmöglichkeit innerhalb eines beschränkten Sinnmenus eingegrenzt wird. Die Sinnfrage kann jedoch auch „Sand im Getriebe" des Systems sein, besonders dann, wenn sie nicht „beantwortet", sondern offengehalten wird (Baumann-Hölzle & Streuli 2009).

Bibliographie

Andrae B (2018) Die Sinne des Lebens: München : Philosophia, [2018]. – 170 Seiten.

Baumann-Hölzle R, Streuli J (2009) Sand oder Öl? – Ethik im Getriebe des Gesundheitswesens. Eine Reflexion über die Rolle der Ethik im Gesundheitswesen und ihr Verhältnis zur Ökonomie. Therapeutische Umschau 66:613 – 616.

Frick E (2019) Kenosis. Eine Sprache für die verborgene Spiritualität finden. In: Frick E, Maidl L (Hg.) Spirituelle Erfahrung in philosophischer Perspektive. Berlin: De Gruyter. 277 – 292.

Hvidt NC (2012) Meaning making and health in contemporary European society. In: Appel K, Danz C, Potz R, Rosenberger S, Walser A (Hg.) Religion in Europe today. Perspectives from social sciences, law, hermeneutics and philosophy of religion. Vienna: Vienna University Press. 173 – 190.

Josuttis M (1974) Der Sinn der Krankheit. Ergebung oder Protest? In: Ds. (Hg.), Praxis des Evangeliums zwischen Politik und Religion. Grundprobleme der praktischen Theologie. München: Kaiser. 117 – 141.

Luhmann N (1990) Der medizinische Code. In: Soziologische Aufklärung 5: Konstruktivistische Perspektiven. Wiesbaden: VS Verlag für Sozialwissenschaften. 183 – 195.

Luhmann N (2002) Die Religion der Gesellschaft. Frankfurt a. M.: Suhrkamp.

Luhmann N (2002/2017) Sinn. In: Baecker D (Hg.), Einführung in die Systemtheorie (Bd. 2). Heidelberg: Carl Auer. 221–246.
Rosa H (2019) „Spirituelle Abhängigkeitserklärung". Die Idee des Mediopassiv als Ausgangspunkt einer radikalen Transformation. In: Dörre K, Rosa H, Becker K, Bose S, Seyd B (Hg.) Große Transformation? Zur Zukunft moderner Gesellschaften: Sonderband des Berliner Journals für Soziologie. Wiesbaden: Springer Fachmedien Wiesbaden. 35–55.
Saake I, Nassehi A, Mayr K (2019) Gegenwarten von Sterbenden. Kölner Zeitschrift für Soziologie und Sozialpsychologie 71:27–52.
Spencer-Brown G (1971) Laws of form. London: Allen and Unwin.
Stein M (2022) The meanings of „meaning". In: Brüntrup G, Frick E (Hg.) Motivation und Sinn. Berlin Boston: De Gruyter [in diesem Band].
Timmins F, Caldeira S (Hg.) (2019) Spirituality in healthcare: Perspectives for innovative practice. Cham: Springer International Publishing.
Vogel R T (2022) Der dunkle Sinn. Die Sinnfrage im Kontext des Schattenkonzepts der Analytischen Psychologie. In: Brüntrup G, Frick E (Hg.) Motivation und Sinn. Berlin Boston: De Gruyter [in diesem Band].

Annette Haußmann

Sinn gesucht

Therapeutische und seelsorgliche Impulse für Spiritual Care angesichts der Sinnfrage

Searching for Meaning?
Therapeutic and Pastoral Impulses for Spiritual Care in the Facing the Question of Meaning

Zusammenfassung: Spiritual Care begleitet Menschen in Lebenssituationen, in denen Sinnfragen aufbrechen sowie Orientierung und Halt gesucht wird. Lebensgeschichtliche Veränderungen können alles Bisherige in Frage stellen und die Zukunft ungewiss erscheinen lassen. Was war, büßt an Gültigkeit und Stabilität ein. Was kommt, verunsichert und fordert zu Neuorientierung und der Suche nach Handlungsalternativen heraus. Zugleich sind Sinn und Spiritualität wichtige Ressourcen, die Menschen in Krisen stabilisieren und Orientierung geben. Aus diesem Grund sind Sinnfragen auch für Spiritual Care enorm wichtig, denn letztere setzt sich zum Ziel, Menschen in Krisen und Umbrüchen therapeutisch, seelsorglich und im Hinblick auf spirituelle Bedürfnisse zu unterstützen. Die Relation von Spiritualität und Sinn wird in ambivalenter Weise zur Grundlage einer flexibel agierenden spirituellen Begleitung, die auch für das Zerbrechliche und Fragmentarische des menschlichen Seins offen ist. Der Beitrag stellt verschiedene Impulse aus Seelsorge und Psychotherapie zum Umgang mit einer spirituellen Sinnsuche vor.

Schlüsselwörter: Seelsorge, Psychotherapie, Sinn, Sinnlosigkeit, Ambivalenz, Hoffnung

Abstract: Spiritual Care provides support for people in life situations in which questions of meaning arise and orientation and stability are sought. Changes in life history can call into question everything that has happened before and make the future seem uncertain. What has been loses its validity and stability. What is to come is unsettling and challenges us to reorient ourselves and search for alternative courses of action. At the same time, meaning and spirituality are important resources that stabilise people in crises and provide orientation. For this reason, questions of meaning are also enormously important for Spiritual Care, which aims to support people in crises and upheavals therapeutically, pastorally, and with regard to spiritual needs. In an ambivalent way, the relationship

https://doi.org/10.1515/9783110787153-004

between spirituality and meaning becomes the basis of a flexibly acting spiritual guidance, which is also open for the fragile and fragmentary nature or human existence. The article presents various impulses from pastoral care and psychotherapy for dealing with a spiritual search for meaning.

Keywords: Pastoral Care, Psychotherapy, meaning, meaninglessness, ambivalence, hope

Die Frage nach dem Sinn – ein interdisziplinäres Unterfangen

> „Die Angst vor der Sinnlosigkeit ist die Angst vor dem Verlust dessen, was uns letztlich angeht, dem Verlust eines Sinnes, der allen Sinngehalten Sinn verleiht. Diese Angst wird durch den Verlust eines geistigen Zentrums erzeugt, durch das Ausbleiben einer Antwort auf die Frage nach dem Sinn der Existenz." (Tillich 2015: 42)

Die Frage nach Sinn durchzieht alle Lebensbereiche und hat tiefgreifende Folgen für den Menschen, sein Wohlbefinden und seine soziale Umwelt. Sie betrifft die Vergangenheit und das Woher des Lebens, ebenso wie die Zukunft und das Wohin im Leben. Meist ist das Leben unbewusst von einem Sinngrund getragen. Seine Bedeutsamkeit und die Sinnhaftigkeit des Ganzen wird erst in Frage gestellt, wenn Sinn nicht mehr selbstverständlich ist, weil das Leben durch Verletzungen zerrüttet wird, Leid und Schwierigkeiten die Gegenwart bestimmen. Doch nicht nur die großen Umbrüche, auch kleine Irritationen im Alltag hinterfragen die Selbstverständlichkeit und verweisen auf die Brüchigkeit von Sinnkonstruktionen und die Kontingenz der Welt. Andererseits kann Sinnerfahrung eine Erfüllung bedeuten, das Leben bereichern, ihm Tiefe, Stabilität und Orientierung verleihen. Sinn ist nie ein leichtfüßiges Gesprächsthema. Wo die Grundfesten des Lebens erschüttert werden, suchen Menschen nach Vergewisserung und Halt, ziehen Selbstverständliches in Zweifel, klagen oder resignieren – eine Herausforderung für alle, die in dieser Situation Begegnung und Begleitung anbieten. Umso relevanter sind Impulse aus Therapie und Seelsorge für Spiritual Care, wenn diese sich als multiprofessionell und interdisziplinär begründete Lebensbegleitung in spirituellen Fragen versteht (Roser 2017; Ständige Konferenz für Seelsorge der EKD 2020).

Sinn hat Konjunktur sowohl in der Seelsorge als auch in der Psychotherapie. John Peteet spricht von einer vierten Welle der „meaning-based psychotherapy", die therapeutisch nicht lediglich auf ein Gesundwerden, sondern auf ein Finden von Bedeutung und Sinn für das gesamte Leben zielt und sich dazu vielfältiger Methoden bedient (Peteet 2018). Das bringt zugleich einen mitunter inflationären

Gebrauch des Sinnbegriffs mit sich, der von der alltagssprachlichen subjektiven Bedeutungszuschreibung über einzelne Lebensziele (Stavemann 2014) und existenzielle Lebensbedeutung (Schnell 2008; Schnell 2020) bis zum Verweis auf einen transzendenten Sinngrund des Seins (Schult 2018) reicht. Sowohl Sinn als auch Spiritualität sind als komplexe multidimensionale Konstrukte zu verstehen, die mit einer Vielzahl von fachlichen Zugängen einhergehen (Kapfhammer 2018) und zu einem Dialog von Psychotherapie, Seelsorge und Spiritual Care anregen (Haußmann & Höfelschweiger 2020).

Zugänge zu Sinn und Spiritualität – und ihre Auswirkung für Spiritual Care

Die Frage nach Sinn ist eng verbunden mit den großen Fragen des Lebens, mit denen sich auch Religion und Spiritualität befassen, die hier synonym komplementär verwendet werden (Zinnbauer & Pargament 2005; Pargament 2013). Wird Sinn in den Rahmen von Spiritual Care gestellt, so muss die Relation von Sinn und Spiritualität geklärt werden. Nach Schnell ist Sinn als multidimensionales Konstrukt mit den Aspekten Kohärenz, Bedeutsamkeit, Orientierung und Zugehörigkeit aufzufassen, wobei Spiritualität eine Facette des Sinns darstellt (Schnell 2020). Umgekehrt kann Sinn auch verstanden werden als ein Aspekt von einer multidimensional angelegten Spiritualität (Pargament 2013). Spiritualität und Sinn werden in den Theoriekonzeptionen unterschiedlich zueinander ins Verhältnis gesetzt, wobei beides miteinander verschmelzen, im Widerspruch stehen oder als Facette des jeweils anderen auftreten kann. Diese komplexe Relation gilt es zu beschreiben und die Konsequenzen für die Möglichkeiten einer begleitenden Spiritual Care auszuloten.

Spiritualität als Sinnerfüllung: Sinnsuche fördern

> „Von Beginn an besteht all das, was Religion ist, darin, den Dingen einen Sinn zu geben.“ (Lacan 2006: 70)

An Religion und Spiritualität wird der Anspruch herangetragen, Sinn zu stiften und eine Antwort auf die Kontingenz des Daseins zu liefern. Auch nach Niklas Luhmann hat Religion die Aufgabe, „die unbestimmbare Welt [...] in eine bestimmbare zu transformieren“ (Luhmann 1977: 26). Anders ausgedrückt: Der Religion wird nicht nur zugetraut, sondern es wird von ihr gefordert, Antworten auf

Sinnfragen zu bieten und dadurch einen stabilen und sinnvollen Rahmen für das Leben zu stiften. Religionspsychologisch werden Spiritualität und Religion als Teil eines Sinnsystems verstanden (Park 2005). Dieses bietet dem Menschen Orientierung und Sicherheit in Stresssituationen und Krisenzeiten und trägt zu deren Bewältigung bei, was zahlreiche empirische Studien belegen (Pargament 1997). Studien aus dem Umfeld der religiösen Coping-Forschung zeigen, wie ein „meaning-based coping" und existenzielle Sinndeutung Menschen in Krisensituationen stärken können, aber auch wie vielschichtig diese Prozesse des Copings sind und dass sie nicht immer linear zu Sinnfindung führen (Pargament 1997). Theologische Perspektiven fokussieren vielfach auf die Verbindung funktionaler und inhaltlicher Definitionen von Religion, indem sie selbige als Möglichkeit für den Umgang mit Kontingenzerleben verstehen. Betont wird eine Ganzheit des Sinns, der nicht identifiziert wird mit einzelnen Lebensbedeutungen von Familie über Arbeit bis Naturerleben (Schnell 2020). Denn Sinn bezieht sich in religiöser Perspektive immer auf einen existenziellen Sinngrund, der die Welt im Innersten zusammenhält, der je nach spiritueller Tradition und religiöser Prägung Gott bzw. das Göttliche genannt wird. Die Erfahrung dieses Sinngrundes ist es, der mit anderen immanenten Formen des Sinns eng verbunden ist und Halt auch im Hereinbrechen der Widerfahrnisse des Lebens verleiht (Gräb 2016). Überträgt man dies auf die Handlungsebene, können Seelsorge und Spiritual Care dazu beitragen, Hilfe zur Sinndeutung zu leisten, Sinndeutungen anzubieten, bei der Sinnsuche auf der Basis spiritueller Grundüberzeugungen zu begleiten (Klessmann 2015). Dabei ist die Überzeugung leitend: „Menschen brauchen Sinn; sie haben das Bedürfnis, die Widerfahrnisse des Lebens in einen Zusammenhang zu bringen, sie nachvollziehbar zu ordnen, sie verstehbar zu machen und damit Ordnung und Kohärenz in ihre Leben zu bringen" (Klessmann 2015: 205).

Spiritualität als Irritation des Sinns: Sinnlosigkeit aushalten

> „In Klage und Verzweiflung liegt mehr ehrliche Hoffnung als in Beteuerung von Sinn und Lebensgewißheit. Trauer hält die Treue zum Anderen, zum Besseren, zum Ende des Leidens, den die Affirmation des Daseins längst verraten hat. Nur wer klagt, hofft." (Luther 1998: 170)

Es gibt andererseits berechtigte Gründe, der Verschmelzung und Identifizierung von Sinn und Spiritualität zu widersprechen. Geht doch Spiritualität keineswegs in der Erfahrung von Sinn und der Konstruktion einer sinnvollen und sinnerfüllten Deutung des Lebens auf. Denn wird Spiritualität als gelebte Religion verstanden, so muss auch die Seite des Lebens, die mit Sinnlosigkeiten und Widersprüchen, mit Widerfahrnissen und Unverfügbarkeit, mit dem Fragmentarischen des Daseins und der Verdunkelung alles Sinnhaften konfrontiert ist, als Teil von Spiritualität begriffen werden. In dieser Sichtweise wird die These, dass Religion dem Leben Sinn verleiht, der fundamentalen Kritik unterzogen. Sinn sei dann gerade nicht in Krankheit und Leiden zu finden, vielmehr müsse solche Sinnlosigkeit als Grunderfahrung des Menschseins ausgehalten werden – auch und gerade von denen, die helfen und unterstützen wollen. Prominent hat diesen Einwand Henning Luther formuliert (Luther 1998; Wagner-Rau 2014). Er hinterfragt, dass Sinn die Leidenden trösten kann, und warnt vor der Verdrängung realer Sinnlosigkeiten: „Trost wird da zur Lüge, wo Sinn suggeriert wird und jeder Anflug eines Verdachts der Unsinnigkeit und Sinnlosigkeit unserer Lebensverhältnisse tabuisiert und verdrängt wird." (Luther 1998: 166 f). Demnach werden Versuche in die Schranken verwiesen, das Leiden unter allen Umständen mit Sinn zu füllen. Die Pointe ist die Perspektive: Dass der einzelne Mensch seinem Leben in Leid und Krankheit Sinn abzugewinnen vermag, darf sein. Aber es ist die von außen zugesprochene Sinnhaftigkeit, die als falscher Trost dort entlarvt wird, wo sie nicht mit der Realität und Deutung des Individuums zusammenpasst. Die Helfenden werden mit ihrer Ohnmacht konfrontiert, die sie gleichzeitig den Leidenden gegenüber zur Solidarität verpflichtet. Isolde Karle unterstreicht dies, indem sie die Seelsorgenden dazu auffordert, Sinnlosigkeit angesichts von Krankheit auszuhalten und ihrer spirituellen Deutung und Aufladung mit Sinn zu widerstehen (Karle 2009). Die Seelsorge hat also angesichts der Sinnfrage eine doppelte Perspektive, indem sie Spiritualität als Ressource anerkennt und fördert, aber einer Verallgemeinerung von Sinn durch spirituelle und religiöse Überzeugungen skeptisch gegenübersteht (Klessmann 2018) und sich nicht ausschließlich als „Sinnlieferantin" versteht (Ziemer 2015: 257 ff). Im Diskurs über Resilienz, erlebte Ohnmacht und Angst gewinnt die Dialektik der Spiritualität zwischen gesundheitsförderlichem Potenzial und notwendiger spiritueller Integration von negativen Gefühlen und Infragestellung von Sinn an Tiefe (Richter 2017).

Spiritual Care zwischen Sinn-Sorge und Sinnlosigkeit: Impulse aus Psychotherapie und Seelsorge

Der Umgang mit Sinn in Spiritual Care kann nur multidimensional verstanden werden und baut auf einem ambivalenten Verhältnis von Sinn und Spiritualität auf. Sinnfragen können nur individuell und innerhalb einer behutsamen Begleitung jenseits von Fremdzuschreibungen bearbeitet werden, daher spreche ich im Folgenden von Impulsen, die zu diesem Prozess einen Beitrag leisten können und flexibel auf die individuelle Situation anzupassen sind.

Identifikation und Konkretion der Sinnfrage zwischen Alltag und Grenzerfahrung

Zunächst ist zu klären, ob und aus welchen Gründen die Sinnfrage gestellt wird, welche Tragweite sie hat und welche Konsequenzen daraus resultieren. Positive Umbrüche wie der Eintritt in eine neue Lebensphase durch Elternschaft, Umzug oder Heirat können genauso Sinnkrisen auslösen wie eine schwere Krankheit, Beziehungskrisen oder der Tod eines geliebten Menschen (Lazarus & Folkman 1984). Auch alltägliche Begebenheiten und kleinere Krisen sind in Betracht zu ziehen, wie etwa Beziehungskonflikte, Einsamkeit oder beruflicher Misserfolg. Im Gespräch kann dann aus einer allgemein gehaltenen Sinnfrage („Alles ist sinnlos“) präzisiert werden, welche Ereignisse dazu geführt haben und mit welchen Gefühlen, Gedanken und Handlungsimpulsen dies korrespondiert. Es geht also weniger um ein allgemeines Philosophieren über Sinnfragen, sondern um eine Verortung im individuellen Erleben und Erleiden. Nicht selten muss die Sinnfrage auch hinter anderen Gefühlen oder Aussagen erst als solche gefunden werden. Sie kann sich hinter Ironie und Sarkasmus, hinter Aggression und Frust oder aber hinter Gleichgültigkeit verbergen. Wird beim aufmerksamen Hören auf Zwischentöne identifiziert, dass es um existenzielle Themen geht, eröffnet sich dadurch eine ganz neue Dimension im Gespräch.

Sinnkrise oder psychische Erkrankung?

Manche Sinnfragen sind Ausdruck von krisenhaften Lebensumbrüchen. Sie können jedoch auch im Rahmen einer psychischen Erkrankung auftreten. Sinnlosigkeit, ein Infragestellen des Bisherigen und ein Sorgen bezüglich des künftigen Lebens sind daher wichtige Indikatoren für eine bestehende psychische Erkrankung. Natürlich sind die Überschneidungsmengen von Krise und manifester psychischer Erkrankung fließend und Sinnfragen sollten keinesfalls vorschnell pathologisiert werden. Das lässt eine Früherkennung entsprechender Hinweise auf eine Erkrankung aber umso wichtiger werden. Nach neueren Erkenntnissen ist das Erleben einer Sinnkrise als relativ unabhängig von gleichzeitig erlebter Sinnerfüllung anzusehen – Sinn und Sinnlosigkeit können also gleichzeitig auftreten (Schnell 2020). Psychopathologisch bedeutsam sind Sinnfragen etwa bei Depression, Suizidalität und Posttraumatischen Belastungsstörungen. Der Verlust von Sinn gehört bei diesen Störungen zum Krankheitsbild und mitunter sind zügige Krisenintervention und Hilfe nötig (Kießling 2018). Bei einer Posttraumatischen Belastungsstörung ist die Zerrüttung des Vertrauens in die Welt angesichts des Erlebten kennzeichnend und das Trauma kann nicht in die Lebensgeschichte integriert werden (Kapfhammer 2018). Sinnlosigkeitsgefühle können ebenso auf Suizidalität hinweisen und müssen unbedingt in ihrer Tiefe und hinsichtlich suizidaler Handlungsimpulse abgeklärt werden. Depression stürzt oftmals in tiefe Sinnfragen und Hoffnungslosigkeit, der Sinnverlust geht also nicht der Erkrankung voraus, sondern ist eines ihrer Kennzeichen. Der Verlust von Spiritualität und Sinn ist häufiges Begleitsymptom von Depression. Gerade für hochreligiöse Menschen ist der Sinnverlust als Glaubensverlust so schmerzlich, weil er den Sinngrund insgesamt fraglich scheinen lässt. Sinnfragen sollten unbedingt ernstgenommen werden, aber es ist nicht zielführend, sie zu vertiefen oder intellektuell zu bearbeiten (Haußmann 2020a; Haußmann 2020c). Gerade Seelsorgende sind für solche Fragen ansprechbar und ermöglichen das Aussprechen von Sinnfragen und integrieren spirituelle Formen wie Rituale, Musik oder religiöse Texte über das Gespräch hinaus. Fallen Sinnverlust und psychische Störung zusammen, insbesondere Depression, PTBS und Suizidalität, ist eine psychotherapeutische Behandlung angezeigt. Eine sorgfältige Diagnostik innerhalb der Therapie, bzw. eine behutsame Erkundung der krankheitsrelevanten Merkmale in der Seelsorge oder Spiritual Care sind deshalb anzuraten. Keineswegs bedeutet es, dass Sinnfragen und Spiritualität ausgeklammert werden. Sie sollten vielmehr in den Behandlungsplan eingebunden werden, denn sie geben Anhaltspunkte dafür, was dem Menschen wichtig und wertvoll ist, aber auch, was ihm im Moment fehlt und wo er sich Veränderung bzw. eine neue Perspektive ersehnt.

Sinnressourcen identifizieren

Die „heilende Kraft des Sinns" (Korsch 2018) wurde in Viktor Frankls Logotherapie, einer Form der humanistisch-existenziell orientierten Psychotherapie, hochgeschätzt. Ihr wurde großes therapeutisches Potenzial und ein wesentlicher Beitrag zur Genesung von psychischer Erkrankung beigemessen (Frankl 1972). Krisen betrachtete Frankl als Anzeichen für ein Defizit von Sinn, die demnach durch die Wiedergewinnung eines persönlichen Lebenssinns behandelt werden. Und in der Tat: Sinn kann in Lebenskrisen und überhaupt für das Leben eine stützende Ressource sein. Daher sind sinnbasierte Interventionen, die auch der Spiritualität neue Impulse geben, eine supportive Ergänzung zur therapeutischen, somatischen und psychischen Behandlung (Mehnert 2006; Mehnert 2010). Das Erleben von Sinnerfüllung als „grundlegende Erfahrung, dass das eigene

Leben sinnhaft und wertvoll ist, dass es sich lohnt, gelebt zu werden“ gründet in einer „Bewertung des eigenen Lebens als kohärent, bedeutsam, orientiert und zugehörig“ (Schnell 2020: 9). Sinn wird dann zur hilfreichen und unterstützenden Ressource, wenn er individuell und konkret auf die jeweilige Lebenssituation bezogen wird. Sinninterventionen bei Krankheit befassen sich deshalb mit der individuellen Zuspitzung der Sinnressourcen (Mehnert 2010; Schnell 2020) und sinnorientierte Therapieformen können das spirituelle Wohlbefinden erhöhen (Breitbart 2017). Wenn mehreren Lebensbereichen von Naturerleben über Selbsterkenntnis bis zum sozialen Engagement Sinn abgewonnen wird, ist eine Sinnorientierung durch ihre Breite besonders tragfähig (Schnell 2020). Bricht eine Säule weg, dann können – zumindest zeitweise – andere Bereiche diese Leerstelle partiell ausgleichen. Sinn ist nicht nur in individualisierter Perspektive unterstützend. Auch spirituelle Tradition und religiöse Gemeinschaft liefern eine Basis im Orientierungssystem, die als sinnstiftend erlebt wird und Coping-Ressourcen zur Verfügung stellt (Pargament 2013). Hierin kann z. B. der Mehrwert von spirituellen Ritualen bestehen, die gerade nicht der individuellen Ausgestaltung bedürfen, sondern in festen Formen und Abläufen, die von der Gemeinschaft getragen und gewährleistet werden, dem Einzelnen Sicherheit und Halt gewähren und stärker in der Leiblichkeit und Emotionalität begründet liegen (Roser 2014; Fries 2017). Darüber hinaus ist aber auch an solche Formen zu denken, die ein konstruktives Nachdenken über Sinn- und Glaubensinhalte in Gemeinschaft ermöglichen, Impulse zu Sinnressourcen geben und ein Ausprobieren von Ressourcen im Alltag anregen.

Lebensgeschichte und Lebensrückblick

Wie die Sinnfrage gestellt wird, wie sie beantwortet wird und welche Perspektiven durch Sinn entstehen, ist rückgebunden an lebensgeschichtliche, soziale und kulturelle Prägungen sowie daraus resultierende Grundannahmen. Populäre Verfahren zur Unterstützung von Sinnfindung und zum Erkunden der Bestandteile eigener Sinnerfüllung sind Lebensrückblickverfahren und narrative Rekonstruktion der Lebensgeschichte (Gräb 1998; Rabaioli-Fischer 2015). Sie sind kurzfristig orientiert oder auf das ganze Leben bezogen (Schnell 2020) und in der Lage, das aufgrund von Krankheit empfundene Leid zu verringern und die Lebensqualität gerade im fortgeschrittenen Alter zu erhöhen (Lan et al. 2017). Die Erzählung liefert hierbei die Chance, sinngebende Elemente aufzuspüren, aber auch die Zusammenhänge, in die das Leben eingebettet ist, neu zu (be)schreiben. Dies kann sowohl im offenen Gespräch geschehen, durch kreatives Schreiben oder aber mit Hilfe von Impulsen durch Kartensets, die Lebensbedeutungen vorgeben (Schnell 2020). Solche Methoden sind immer als Anregungen eines Prozesses zu sehen, der sich außerhalb der Interventionen im Alltag fortsetzt. Die lebensgeschichtliche Narration hat im Zusammenhang mit Traumata eine wichtige Bedeutung erlangt. Hier dient das Erzählen der Rekonstruktion und der Einbettung in kognitive Strukturen und wird therapeutisch und seelsorglich zur Verarbeitung von emotionaler Übererregung und Spannungszuständen genutzt (Kapfhammer 2018; Schult 2020). Auch in der Seelsorge hat die Erzählung von Lebensgeschichte eine zentrale Bedeutung. Hier wird sie als Möglichkeit religiös-spiritueller Selbst- und Lebensdeutung angesehen, die nicht nur auf Selbsterkenntnis und Sinnschöpfung zielt, sondern im Verweis auf einen tieferen Seinsgrund ein „Gegründet- und Gehaltensein" findet (Gräb 1998: 67). Zugleich ist die Brüchigkeit, Vorläufigkeit und Fragmentarität ebenso zur Lebensgeschichte gehörig und verweist auf die Notwendigkeit der wiederholten Erzählung, der Selbstvergewisserung und das durch Spiritualität auch in Unruhe gehaltene Dasein (Luther 1998). Solche Brüche in der Lebensgeschichte bergen immer auch die Chance zu einer neuen Erzählung, die das Alte nicht lediglich vergewissernd wiederholt, und sind darum als Wandel im besten Sinn zu verstehen (Roessler 2016). Durch Spiritual Care können spirituelle und religiöse Prägungen, Erlebnisse und Sinn-Ressourcen gezielt in die Narration von Lebensgeschichte eingebunden werden.

Wenn Sinn belastet

Sinn motiviert: Wer in seinem Tun und Lassen einen Sinn sieht, verhält sich trotz Krankheit, Widerständen und Stress gesundheitsförderlicher und achtet mehr auf sich (Schnell 2020). Und Sinn belastet: Denn Sinn kann auch in schädlicher Weise Menschen über die Belastungsgrenzen hinaus dazu motivieren, ihr bisheriges Verhalten aufrecht zu erhalten. Diese Beobachtung lässt sich etwa in der Pflege von Angehörigen machen, wenn die häusliche Pflege trotz hoher Belastungsreaktionen der Pflegenden weitergeführt wird, weil sie im individuellen Erleben Sinn macht, obwohl sie zugleich belastet – eine hochgradig ambivalente Situation (Haußmann 2019). Insbesondere wenn Sinn durch ein religiös-spirituelles Orientierungs- und Bedeutungssystem getragen ist, kommt es mitunter zu solchen Überlastungen. Diese sind für therapeutische und seelsorgliche Begleitung unbedingt mit im Blick zu halten, da Sinn unter diesen Umständen auch zur Belastung beitragen oder zur Belastung werden kann. Gerade für hochreligiöse Menschen lässt sich auch empirisch zeigen, dass diese einerseits von einer stabilen Sinnorientierung als Ressource profitieren, aber auch Zweifel, Anfechtung und Ärger im spirituellen Rahmen erleben (Exline et al. 2012). Vorübergehende

Sinnlosigkeit ist auch eine spirituelle Herausforderung, die Gefühle von Leere und Erschöpfung nach sich zieht (Sautermeister et al. 2017). Behutsam gilt es in Spiritual Care, solche Zusammenhänge zwischen Sinn und Spiritualität transparent zu machen, gegebenenfalls zu hinterfragen und mit anderen religiösen und sinnhaften Überzeugungen ins Gespräch zu bringen (Haußmann 2016). Die Ambivalenz zwischen Fürsorge und Selbstschutz gilt überdies für die Akteur-/innen im Bereich Spiritual Care: Das helfende, unterstützende Tun wird einerseits als sinnhaft erfahren, kann jedoch angesichts schwieriger Begegnungen oder schwer auszuhaltender Konflikte auch belastend sein (Kunz 2018). Supervision ist in solchen Zusammenhängen eine förderliche und notwendige Ergänzung für spirituell Begleitende (Weiß 2011). Zu berücksichtigen sind auch spirituelle Konflikte, wenn der Sinn des Ganzen brüchig wird, die emotional sehr belasten und eine zusätzliche Bürde zu den Lebensereignissen aufladen können (Exline 2013). Solcher „Sinnschmerz“ als ein Leiden an Spiritualität, die nicht (mehr) trägt, fordert Spiritual Care heraus (Peng-Keller 2017). Manche Menschen deuten Widerfahrnisse wie Krankheit im Rahmen ihrer Spiritualität als göttliche Aufgabe (Fitchett et al. 2014), sie suchen Sinn im posttraumatischen Wachstum (Exline et al. 2017) oder bewerten ihr Leiden als spirituellen Auftrag. Solche Sinndeutungen führen mitunter zu einer Vertiefung des Leidens oder zu einem passiven Aushalten der Situation und sind deshalb in der Begleitung sensibel wahrzunehmen, auf ihre Implikationen hin zu befragen und evtl. dort zur Transformation anzuregen, wo sich die Überzeugungen nicht als lebensdienlich erweisen (Pargament 2007; Haußmann 2019).

Sinnlosigkeit aushalten

Wenn Sinn abhandenkommt, kann dies einerseits als Chance erlebt werden, löst aber auch großes Leid aus. Von Sinnlosigkeit sind dann auch die Helfenden in Spiritual Care selbst betroffen. Sich mit dem Warum des anderen Menschen, seinem Leiden am fehlenden Sinn zu konfrontieren, löst Impulse aus, Sinn wiederherstellen oder dabei unterstützen zu wollen, statt passiv bleiben zu müssen. Diese Ohnmacht auszuhalten, kann daher ein wichtiger Baustein in der Begleitung bei Sinnverlust sein. Es ist ein stilles Gegenstück zum Aktionismus des Helfens, ein Da-Sein („being-there“) und Mit-Sein („being-with“) (Nolan 2011), das die Leere der Sinnfrage auszuhalten bereit ist und für eine spirituelle Präsenz offenhält. Sinn lässt sich nur begrenzt konstruktiv herstellen, er lässt sich nicht von außen aufzeigen. Sinnerfüllung ereignet sich und bleibt letztlich unverfügbar. In der Palliativbegleitung oder im Krankenhaus in schwerer Krankheit, bei nahendem Tod ist die Sorge um spirituelle Bedürfnisse angesichts von Schmerz und

Abschied eine wichtige Komponente der Begleitung, die als gemeinsames Wachen („Watch with me“) verstanden werden kann (Saunders 2005; Chilian 2020). Die seelsorgliche Betonung des Aushaltens hat ihre Berechtigung (Karle 2009) und wehrt einer ausschließlichen Identifizierung von Spiritual Care mit Sinn-Sorge – wenn auch die Haltung unbedingt von passiver Resignation unterschieden werden muss.

Sinnfindung als dialogische Auseinandersetzung

Wenn überhaupt, so kann ein Mensch seinen Lebenssinn nur selbst finden, von außen kann Sinn nicht vermittelt werden. Zugleich ist aber die soziale Dimension jeder Sinnsuche wesentlich. Denn nicht nur in der individuellen Auseinandersetzung stellen sich Sinnfragen, sondern diese werden im Gespräch, in der konstruktiven Bearbeitung im sozialen Kontext, im Miteinander und in der Gemeinschaft bearbeitet. Insofern kann Spiritual Care dazu anregen, solchen Austausch zu Sinn und Spiritualität zu fördern, und damit einen Beitrag zu einer sorgenden Gemeinschaft leisten (Frick & Roser 2011; Haußmann 2020b). Pointiert formuliert ginge es dann nicht etwa um *Antworten* auf die Sinnfrage, sondern darum, Anregungen und Impulse für die *Suche* nach Antworten darauf anzubieten, wann und auf welche Weise eine Beschäftigung mit dem Sinn des Lebens sinnvoll und lebensdienlich ist – und wann nicht. So kann sich ein neuer Blick auf das Leben eröffnen. Es ginge dann weder um eine Hilfe zum Sinn noch um eine Anleitung zur Sinnfindung, sondern um die Begleitung angesichts von Sinnfragen und eine ressourcenorientierte Einbindung von allem, was diesen Prozess förderlich unterstützt. Ähnlich kann Spiritualität als Ressource für Suchende differenziert und am Individuum, seiner Lebensgeschichte und sozialen Einbindung orientiert in den seelsorglichen bzw. therapeutischen Prozess einbezogen werden. Spirituelle Impulse sind vielseitig und können die sprachliche Dimension auch durch Rituale, Symbole, Stille oder Bilder überschreiten, was die Sinnsuche wohltuend nicht allein auf die kognitive Dimension festlegt (Haußmann 2021).

Jenseits des Sinns: Gleichgültigkeit, Hoffnung und Versenkung

Existenzielle Indifferenz

Während Frankl annahm, dass allen Menschen ein universaler Wille zum Sinn innewohne und ein Mangel daran zu einer „noogenen Neurose" führen müsse (Frankl 1972), zeigen Studien heute, dass fehlender Sinn nicht zwangsläufig ein Indiz für eine Störung ist. Manche Menschen brauchen und suchen keinen Sinn. Sie stehen der Sinnfrage unentschlossen oder gleichgültig gegenüber und zeigen keine Anzeichen einer Krise (Schnell 2010). Die Gründe dafür sind vielschichtig, wobei das Phänomen in den letzten Jahren abnimmt, da junge Menschen wieder stärker an Sinn- und Zukunftsfragen interessiert sind. Ein deutlicher Zusammenhang zeigt sich zur Spiritualität: Wer Lebensbedeutungen von Spiritualität, Religiosität, Fürsorge, Generativität, Harmonie, Gemeinschaft und bewusstem Erleben zustimmt, ist wenig indifferent (Schnell 2020). Indifferenz ist bedeutsam für eine sinnsensible Spiritual Care, denn sie kann auch als Indiz für geringe Selbstwirksamkeit, Bindungsvermeidung durch sozialen Rückzug, Einsamkeit und Resignation gewertet werden (Schnell 2020).

Hoffnung und Sehnsucht

Angesichts der Verletzlichkeit menschlichen Lebens kann es in theologischer und religiöser Hinsicht keine Perspektive sein, dem Leben in jeder Hinsicht einen Sinn abzuringen. In Krankheit, Leiden und Tod geht es weniger darum, diesen Lebensereignissen Sinn zuzuschreiben, sondern dem Schmerz Ausdruck zu verleihen und die Sehnsucht nach einer Veränderung offenzuhalten (Luther 1987). Es macht dabei einen wesentlichen Unterschied, ob dem Erleiden selbst Sinn zugesprochen wird, oder trotz des Hereinbrechens solcher Erfahrungen an einem sinnhaften Daseinsgrund oder einer religiös-spirituellen Orientierung festgehalten wird. Hoffnung wird dann zum Gegenbegriff für Sinn und Leitmetapher für das Religiöse (Luther 1998). Sie hält offen, dass noch etwas aussteht, dass die Welt, so wie sie ist und erlebt wird, nicht in letzter Konsequenz kohärent und sinnhaft ist. Abgründe und Leid sind ein faktischer Bestandteil der Welt, gegen die es aus Perspektive des Glaubens zu protestieren gilt. In der christlichen Tradition steht für diesen Protest gegen den Tod das Kreuz, Symbol für das Leiden, die dunkle Nacht (Pfeifer 2018), auf deren letztliche Überwindung wir hoffen.

Wenn Spiritual Care den Aspekt des Hoffens und der Sehnsucht integriert, erweitert sich der Spiritualitätsbegriff und sorgt für mehr Ambivalenztoleranz, statt Aspekten einer rein ressourcenorientierten positiven Psychologie Vorschub zu leisten (Klessmann 2018; Haußmann 2019).

Meditation, Achtsamkeit und Gebet: Vom Leben im Moment

Sinnfragen fokussieren weite Zeiträume in der Vergangenheit durch die Erörterung von Lebensgeschichte oder weisen über die Gegenwart hinaus auf die künftige Gestaltung des Lebens hin. Demgegenüber bietet Achtsamkeit eine Haltung an, wie ein Mensch im Moment verweilen kann und regt dazu an, weniger kognitiv zu überlegen, sondern auf aktuelle Gefühle zu horchen, während Gedanken kommen und gehen dürfen (Heidenreich & Michalak 2013). Achtsamkeit hat sich als Antigrübelstrategie bei Depression und Ängsten bewährt und kann von allzu drängenden Sinnfragen ablenken bzw. den Sinn im Kleinen, im Erleben von Stille und Alltag finden (Michalak et al. 2018). Dieses Leben im Moment, eine angeregte Konzentration auf die kleinen Dinge des Lebens, die vermeintliche Alltäglichkeit, kann die Dankbarkeit für kleine Momente fördern (Freund & Lehr 2019), statt an den großen Fragen der Existenz zu (ver)zweifeln. Auch Meditation regt zu einer Konzentration auf das Jetzt an und gibt darüber hinaus dem Hören, der Stille und dem Empfangen Raum (Wachholtz & Austin 2013; Kabat-Zinn & Kierdorf 2015). Gebet ist eine weitere Möglichkeit, Sinnfragen zu äußern, zu klagen und erlebte Sinnlosigkeit in den größeren Kontext der Spiritualität und Transzendenz zu stellen (Baumann 2017). Gebet drängt auf Resonanz und nimmt auch Erfahrungen von Menschen auf, die keinen Sinn finden, Leid erleben, aber keine Antworten hören oder vergeblich auf Heilung und Hilfe warten (Kunz 2017). Indem das Gebet solchen Erfahrungen innerhalb der Spiritualität einen Platz einräumt, eröffnet es Raum für spirituelles Leben in Krankheit und Gesundheit, das nicht auf Sinnerfüllung drängt, sondern Stärkung jenseits der Funktionalisierung von Religion und Spiritualität sucht.

Spiritual Care mit Sensibilität für Ambivalenz und Prozesshaftigkeit von Sinnsuche

Beide Pole der Spiritualität, ihre Resonanz auf Sinnlosigkeit und Sinnfragen sowie ihr Potenzial zur Sinngebung und Sinnerfüllung sind für Spiritual Care bedeutsam und müssen in einer dynamischen Spannung zueinander gesehen werden. Eine Integration dieser spannungsreichen Ambivalenz führt zu einer Berücksichtigung der Ressourcen *und* des Belastungspotenzials von Spiritualität. Die Frage nach dem Sinn lässt sich weder allgemeingültig noch erschöpfend klären. Vielmehr scheinen Sinnfragen prozesshaft in spezifischen Lebenssituationen immer neu auf, werden bearbeitet, wieder losgelassen, ordnen sich neu, weitere Aspekte ergänzen sich, das Leben selbst bringt durch seine Ereignisse wieder Sinn durcheinander oder erneute Ordnung in das Bestehende. Selbes gilt für Spiritualität, die sich im Lauf des Lebens in einem dynamischen Prozess spiegelt, in dessen Verlauf Überzeugungen und Prägungen, Gefühle und Gedanken immer wieder dem Wandel unterzogen sind (Haußmann 2019). Die Suche nach Sinn ist demnach nicht abgeschlossen, sondern ihr liegt zugrunde, dass sie sich stets neu formiert und damit Spiritualität und Religiosität lebendig erhält (Pargament 2007). Sorge um den Sinn angesichts der lebensgeschichtlichen Zumutungen von Krankheit und Endlichkeit kann dann vielfaches bedeuten: Sinnsuche unterstützen, Sinnlosigkeit aushalten, gegen Resignation und Depression kämpfen und die Hoffnung aufrechterhalten (Klessmann 2016). Eine Sorge um die spirituelle Dimension des Menschseins, die als multiprofessionelle Spiritual Care Sinnsuchende unterstützen will, sollte sich demnach als Prozessbegleitung oder Begegnungsmöglichkeit auf diesem Weg der Suche verstehen, wenn sie dem Transformativen Raum geben will. Sinnsuche findet nicht im luftleeren Raum statt, sie kann sich bestehender Traditionen, Bilder, Symbole und Geschichten bedienen, die einen überindividuellen Rahmen stiften und Suchprozesse des Einzelnen anregen. Andererseits ist Spiritual Care offen für spirituelle Konflikte, Sinnlosigkeit und Brüche des Lebens. Dazu benötigt es die Perspektive mehrerer Disziplinen und Professionen im Rahmen von „Spiritual Care im Plural“ (Peng-Keller 2015; Frick & Peng-Keller 2017), die sich als bewusst vielstimmig auf den Sinn Bezug nehmendes Unterstützungsnetz versteht. Sinn ist in spiritueller Hinsicht auch ein Beziehungsbegriff. Sinnsuche ereignet sich in spiritueller Gemeinschaft, im Rückgriff auf gegebene Traditionen, in Auseinandersetzung im zwischenmenschlichen Gespräch. Spiritual Care lädt dazu ein: Das eigene Leben entdecken, trotz seiner Brüche oder gerade angesichts der Brüche und der Unverfügbarkeit des Lebens, das es zu gestalten gilt. Sinnsuche bedeutet auch, einer nicht nur selbst hergestellten, aktiv konstruierten, sondern einer sich ereignenden Sinnhaftigkeit des eigenen Lebens auf der Spur zu bleiben. In dieser Hoffnungsperspektive begleitet Spiritual Care Sinnsuchende, Sinnzweifelnde und Sinnerfüllte angesichts der großen und kleinen Lebensereignisse.

Literatur

Baumann K (2017) Gebet in schwerer Krankheit und Spiritual Care: Zwischen Sinnsuche, Klage und Akzeptanz des Unverständlichen. In: Peng-Keller S, Beintker M, Eurich J, Thomas G, Welker M, Tietz C (Hg.) Gebet als Resonanzereignis: Annäherungen im Horizont von Spiritual Care. Gottingen: Vandenhoeck & Ruprecht. 143–158.
Breitbart W (Hg.) (2017) Meaning-centered psychotherapy in the cancer setting: Finding meaning and hope in the face of suffering. New York: Oxford University Press.
Chilian L (2020) „Watch with me". Wege zum Menschen 72:408–419.
Exline J (2013) Religious and Spiritual Struggles. In: Pargament KI (Hg.) APA Handbook of Psychology, Religion, and Spirituality: Volume 1: Context, Theory, and Research. Washington D.C: American Psychological Association. 459–475.
Exline J, Hall T, Pargament KI, Harriott V (2017) Predictors of growth from spiritual struggle among Christian undergraduates: Religious coping and perceptions of helpful action by God are both important. The Journal of Positive Psychology 12:501–508.
Exline J, Kaplan K, Grubbs J (2012) Anger, exit, and assertion: Do people see protest toward God as morally acceptable? Psychology of Religion and Spirituality 4:264–277.
Fitchett G, Winter-Pfändler U, Pargament K I (2014) Struggle with the divine in swiss patients visited by chaplains: Prevalence and correlates. Journal of Health Psychology 19:966–976.
Frankl V (1972) Der Wille zum Sinn: Ausgewählte Vorträge über Logotherapie. Bern: Huber.
Freund H, Lehr D (2019) Dankbarkeit in der Psychotherapie: Ressource und Herausforderung. Göttingen: Hogrefe Verlag.
Frick E, Peng-Keller S (2017) „Spiritual Care" im Plural: Editorial. Spiritual Care 6:151–152.
Frick E, Roser T (Hg.) (2011) Spiritualität und Medizin: Gemeinsame Sorge um den kranken Menschen. Stuttgart: Kohlhammer Verlag.
Fries T (2017) Raum, Leib und Ritualität. Beobachtungen zu einigen Aspekten verleiblichter Spiritualität in Schweizer Universitätsspitälern. Spiritual Care 6:153–165.
Gräb W (1998) Lebensgeschichten, Lebensentwürfe, Sinndeutungen: Eine praktische Theologie gelebter Religion. Gütersloh: Kaiser Gütersloher Verlags-Haus.
Gräb W (2016) Religion als individuelle Erfahrung von Sinn. In: Kühnlein M (Hg.) Gott und Sinn: Im interdisziplinären Gespräch mit Volker Gerhardt. : 65–77.
Haußmann A (2016) 4.7 Wege zur Veränderung – Motivierende Gesprächsführung. In: Hax-Schoppenhorst T, Jünger S, Arlt S (Hg.) Das Depressions-Buch für Pflege- und Gesundheitsberufe: Menschen mit Depressionen gekonnt pflegen und behandeln. Bern: Hogrefe. 267–279.
Haußmann A (2019) Ambivalenz und Dynamik: Eine empirische Studie zu Religion in der häuslichen Pflege. Berlin, Boston: de Gruyter.
Haußmann A (2020a) Depression and Spirituality/Religion: An Ambivalent Relationship. In: Jakob B, Weyel B (Hg.) Spirituality, Mental Health, and Social Support: A Community Approach. Berlin: de Gruyter. 56–89.
Haußmann A (2020b) Füreinander sorgen. Soziale Unterstützung für pflegende Angehörige und die Bedeutung Sorgender Gemeinschaften. Spiritual Care 10:74–85.
Haußmann A (2020c) Suche nach Spiritualität und Sinn bei Depression. Was können Seelsorge und Kognitive Verhaltenstherapie voneinander lernen? In: Haußmann A, Höfelschweiger R

(Hg.) Spiritualität und Sinn: Seelsorge und Kognitive Verhaltenstherapie im Dialog. Leipzig: Evangelische Verlagsanstalt.
Haußmann A (2021) Die Kraft der Bilder. Visuelle Kommunikation in sozialen Medien und ihre Potenziale für Spiritual Care und Seelsorge. Spiritual Care: aop.
Haußmann A, Höfelschweiger R (Hg.) (2020) Spiritualität und Sinn: Seelsorge und Kognitive Verhaltenstherapie im Dialog. Leipzig: Evangelische Verlagsanstalt.
Heidenreich T, Michalak J (Hg.) (2013) Die ‚dritte Welle' der Verhaltenstherapie: Grundlagen und Praxis. Weinheim: Beltz.
Kabat-Zinn J, Kierdorf T (2015) Im Alltag Ruhe finden: Meditationen für ein gelassenes Leben. München: Knaur.
Kapfhammer H-P (2018) Sinn – eine empirisch belastbare Kategorie in Psychiatrie und Psychotherapie? Das Beispiel traumatischer Erfahrungen – zwischen seelischer Erschütterung, körperlicher Beschädigung, Resilienz und persönlichem Wachstum. In: Korsch D (Hg.) Die heilende Kraft des Sinns: Viktor E. Frankl in philosophischer, theologischer und therapeutischer Betrachtung. Stuttgart: Kohlhammer Verlag. 103–139.
Karle I (2009) Sinnlosigkeit aushalten!: Ein Plädoyer gegen die Spiritualisierung von Krankheit. Wege zum Menschen 61:19–34.
Kießling K (2018) Psychiatrische Notfälle und psychische Krisen in der Seelsorge – am Beispiel von depressiven Erkrankungen und Ängsten. In: Sautermeister J, Skuban T (Hg.) Handbuch psychiatrisches Grundwissen für die Seelsorge. Freiburg, Basel, Wien: Verlag Herder. 34–53.
Klessmann M (2015) Seelsorge: Begleitung, Begegnung, Lebensdeutung im Horizont des christlichen Glaubens. Ein Lehrbuch. Neukirchen-Vluyn: Neukirchener Theologie.
Klessmann M (2016) Seelsorge im Krankheitsfall. In: Engemann W (Hg.) Handbuch der Seelsorge: Grundlagen und Profile. Leipzig: Evangelische Verlagsanstalt. 491–513.
Klessmann M (2018) Ambivalenz und Glaube: Warum sich in der Gegenwart Glaubensgewissheit zu Glaubensambivalenz wandeln muss. Stuttgart: Kohlhammer Verlag.
Korsch D (Hg.) (2018) Die heilende Kraft des Sinns: Viktor E. Frankl in philosophischer, theologischer und therapeutischer Betrachtung. Stuttgart: Kohlhammer Verlag.
Kunz R (2017) Beten in der Anfechtung: Praktisch-theologische Annäherungen an Gebete, die nicht auf Resonanz stoßen. In: Peng-Keller S, Beintker M, Eurich J, Thomas G, Welker M, Tietz C (Hg.) Gebet als Resonanzereignis: Annäherungen im Horizont von Spiritual Care. Gottingen: Vandenhoeck & Ruprecht. 159–176.
Kunz R (2018) Dem Herrn sei's geklagt. In: Kreitzscheck D, Springhart H (Hg.) Geschichten vom Leben: Zugänge zur Theologie der Seelsorge. Festschrift für Wolfgang Drechsel. Leipzig: Evangelische Verlagsanstalt.
Lacan J (2006) Der Triumph der Religion welchem vorausgeht der Diskurs an die Katholiken. Wien: Turia + Kant.
Lan X, Xiao H, Chen Y (2017) Effects of life review interventions on psychosocial outcomes among older adults: A systematic review and meta-analysis. Geriatrics & gerontology international 17:1344–1357.
Lazarus R S, Folkman S (1984) Stress, appraisal, and coping. New York, N.Y.: Springer.
Luhmann N (1977) Funktion der Religion. Frankfurt a. M.: Suhrkamp.
Luther H (1987) Schmerz und Sehnsucht: Praktische Theologie in der Mehrdeutigkeit des Alltags. Theologia practica 22:295–317.

Luther H (1998) Die Lügen der Tröster: Das Beunruhigende des Glaubens als Herausforderung für die Seelsorge. Praktische Theologie 33:163–176.
Mehnert A (2006) Sinnfindung und Spiritualitat bei Patienten mit chronischen korperlichen Erkrankungen. Bundesgesundheitsblatt, Gesundheitsforschung, Gesundheitsschutz 49:780–787.
Mehnert A (2010) Sinnbasierte Interventionen. In: Diegelmann C, Isermann M (Hg.) Ressourcenorientierte Psychoonkologie: Psyche und Körper ermutigen. Stuttgart: Kohlhammer Verlag. 127–133.
Michalak J, Meibert P, Heidenreich T (2018) Achtsamkeit üben: Hilfe bei Stress, Depression, Ängsten und häufigem Grübeln. Göttingen: Hogrefe.
Nolan S (2011) Spiritual care at the end of life: The chaplain as a „hopeful presence". London, Philadelphia: Jessica Kingsley Publishers.
Pargament KI (1997) The Psychology of Religion and Coping: Theory, research, practice. New York NY u. a.: Guilford Press.
Pargament KI (2007) Spiritually integrated psychotherapy: Understanding and addressing the sacred. New York: Guilford Press.
Pargament KI (2013) Searching for the sacred: Toward a nonreductionistic theory of spirituality. In: Pargament KI, Exline J, Jones J (Hg.) APA handbook of psychology, religion, and spirituality (Vol 1): Context, theory, and research. Washington: American Psychological Association. 257–273.
Park C (2005) Religion as Meaning-Making Framework in Coping with Life Stress. Journal of Social Issues 61:707–729.
Peng-Keller S (2015) Spiritual Care als theologische Herausforderung: Eine Ortsbestimmung. Theologische Literaturzeitung 140:454–467.
Peng-Keller S (2017) Spiritual Pain. Annäherung an einen Schlüsselbegriff interprofessioneller Spiritual Care. Spiritual Care 6:295–302.
Peteet J (2018) A fourth wave of psychotherapies: Moving beyond recovery toward well-being. Harvard review of psychiatry 26:90–95.
Pfeifer S (2018) Seelenfinsternis und dunkle Nacht der Seele – Depression und Spiritualität. In: Utsch M, Bonelli RM, Pfeifer S (Hg.) Psychotherapie und Spiritualität: Mit existenziellen Konflikten und Transzendenzfragen professionell umgehen. Berlin: Springer. 143–153.
Rabaioli-Fischer B (2015) Biografisches Arbeiten und Lebensrückblick in der Psychotherapie: Ein Praxishandbuch. Göttingen: Hogrefe.
Richter C (2017) Ohnmacht und Angst aushalten: Kritik der Resilienz in Theologie und Philosophie. Stuttgart: Kohlhammer Verlag.
Roessler I (2016) Krise, Trauma und Konflikt als Ausgangspunkte der Seelsorge. In: Engemann W (Hg.) Handbuch der Seelsorge: Grundlagen und Profile. Leipzig: Evangelische Verlagsanstalt. 451–475.
Roser T (2014) Praktische Theologie] Schmerz ausdrücken und behandeln in Ritualen. Praktische Theologie 49:221–227.
Roser T (2017) Spiritual Care: Der Beitrag von Seelsorge zum Gesundheitswesen.
Saunders C (2005) Watch with me: Inspiration for a life in hospice care. Lancaster: Observatory Publications.
Sautermeister J, Frick E, Büssing A, Baumann K (2017) Wenn die Sinnquelle zu versiegen droht. Spiritual Care 6:197–207.

Schnell T (2008) Implizite Religiosität. In: Gräb W (Hg.) Individualisierung – Spiritualität – Religion: Transformationsprozesse auf dem religiösen Feld in interdisziplinärer Perspektive. Berlin, Münster: Lit. 111–135.
Schnell T (2010) Existential Indifference: Another Quality of Meaning in Life. Journal of Humanistic Psychology 50:351–373.
Schnell T (2020) Psychologie des Lebenssinns. Berlin, Germany: Springer.
Schult M (2018) Sinnfragen in der Seelsorg: Viktor E. Frankl als Impulsgeber der Poimenik. In: Korsch D (Hg.) Die heilende Kraft des Sinns: Viktor E. Frankl in philosophischer, theologischer und therapeutischer Betrachtung. Stuttgart: Kohlhammer Verlag. 83–101.
Schult M (2020) Für Sinn sorgen? Seelsorge und kognitive Verhaltenstherapie nach traumatischen Ereignissen. In: Haußmann A, Höfelschweiger R (Hg.) Spiritualität und Sinn: Seelsorge und Kognitive Verhaltenstherapie im Dialog. Leipzig: Evangelische Verlagsanstalt. 139–162.
Ständige Konferenz für Seelsorge der EKD (2020) Seelsorgliche Spiritual Care als kirchlicher Beitrag im Gesundheitswesen. Hannover.
Stavemann H (2014) Lebenszielanalyse und Lebenszielplanung: In Therapie und Beratung. Weinheim, Basel: Beltz, PVU.
Tillich P (2015) Der Mut zum Sein. Berlin/Boston: de Gruyter.
Wachholtz A, Austin E (2013) Contemporary spiritual meditation: Practices and outcomes. In: Pargament KI, Exline J, Jones J (Hg.) APA handbook of psychology, religion, and spirituality (Vol 1): Context, theory, and research. Washington: American Psychological Association. 311–327.
Wagner-Rau U (2014) Seelsorge als religiöse Praxis: Überlegungen im Gespräch mit Henning Luther. In: Fechtner K, Mulia C (Hg.) Henning Luther: Impulse für eine Praktische Theologie der Spätmoderne. Stuttgart: Kohlhammer. 127–140.
Weiß H (2011) Seelsorge – Supervision – Pastoralpsychologie. Neukirchen-Vluyn: Neukirchener Theologie.
Ziemer J (2015) Seelsorgelehre. Stuttgart, Göttingen: UTB GmbH; Vandenhoeck & Ruprecht.
Zinnbauer B, Pargament KI (2005) Religiousness and spirituality. In: Paloutzian R, Park C (Hg.) Handbook of the Psychology of Religion and Spirituality. Princeton, N.J.: Recording for the Blind & Dyslexic. 21–42.

Florian Lampersberger

Der Sinn der Sinnfrage

Sprachphilosophische und psychoanalytische Zugänge

The Meaning of the Question of Meaning
Perspectives from Philosophy of Language and Psychoanalysis

Zusammenfassung: Im Folgenden wird versucht, den Sinn der Sinnfrage durch Zuhilfenahme sprachphilosophischer und psychoanalytischer Konzepte besser zu verstehen. Zunächst ergibt die Untersuchung des Alltagsgebrauchs der Sinn-Frage, dass man als Fragestellender nicht auf konkrete Tatsachen aus ist, sondern vielmehr Antworten darauf sucht, was ein wertvolles Leben konstituiert. Was genau man unter dem Sinn-Begriff verstehen kann, wird durch Ordnung des semantischen Feldes um Sinn genauer betrachtet. Durch Differenzierung der Facetten von Sinnhaftigkeit und Abgrenzung von Sinnfremdem und Sinnfreiem werden im nächsten Schritt Bedingungen dafür deutlich, wie Leben überhaupt Träger von Sinn sein kann. Daraufhin werden verschiedene Ebenen des Sinnvollseins untersucht – vom Sinn einer Handlung bis zum Sinn des Kosmos – und zwischen Sinn im Leben und Sinn des Lebens unterschieden. Die Begründungszusammenhänge werden anschließend anhand gängiger Sinn-Konzeptionen aufgefächert, wobei die zwischen subjektivem und objektivem Naturalismus liegende Hybrid-Theorie Susan Wolfs genauer betrachtet wird. Im Anschluss werden die Entwicklungsbedingungen für Sinn-Erleben anhand psychischer Ich-Fähigkeiten zu Symbolisierung, Mentalisierung und libidinöser Besetzung dargestellt. Zuletzt werden im verdeckten Symptom-Sinn Sinn-destruktive Seiten des unbewussten Seelenlebens aufgedeckt, aber auch Sinn-ermöglichende Aspekte aufgefunden. Damit wird deutlich, dass die Psychoanalyse entgegen der Vorwürfe sinnzentrierter Psychotherapieschulen (insbesondere der Logotherapie) Wichtiges zur Sinn-Frage beisteuern und in der Sinn-Kontroverse ein Versöhnungsangebot unterbreiten kann.

Schlüsselwörter: Sinn-Begriff / Sinn-Positionen / Sinn-Fähigkeit / Objektbeziehungstheorie / Sinn-Unbewusstes

Abstract: The author attempts to uncover the meaning of the question of meaning through philosophy of language and psychoanalysis. The investigation of how the question of meaning is used in ordinary language shows that one is not looking for facts but rather for answers about the constitution of a valuable

https://doi.org/10.1515/9783110787153-005

life. It becomes apparent that an intended non-answerability in asking the question of meaning expresses personal distress. How to understand the term of meaning is examined more closely by exploring the semantic field around meaning. By differentiating between the facets of meaning and the demarcation between 'meaning-external' and 'nonsensical', conditions become clear for how life can be a carrier of meaning. Hereupon different levels of meaningfulness are examined and a distinction is made between meaning in life and meaning of life. Afterwards, the explanatory connections are fanned out using common concepts of meaning, with Susan Wolf's theory being picked out. Subsequently, the developmental conditions for experiencing meaning are presented on the basis of psychological ego-abilities for symbolisation, mentalisation and libidinous cathexis. Lastly, the hidden meaning of symptoms reveals a meaning-destructive side, but also aspects that enable meaning. Thus it shows, an offer of peace is made in the controversy between meaning centered psychotherapy (especially logotherapy) and psychoanalysis.

Keywords: Notion of meaning / positions of meaning / capacity of meaning / object relation theory / unconscious meaning

> „[...] hast du ... äh, das heißt ..."
> „Eine Antwort für euch?", unterbrach Deep Thought würdevoll. „Ja, die habe ich."
> Die beiden Männer zitterten vor froher Erwartung. Ihr Warten war nicht vergeblich gewesen.
> „Es gibt tatsächlich eine?", hauchte Phouchg.
> „Es gibt tatsächlich eine", bestätigte Deep Thought.
> „Auf alles? Auf die Große Frage nach dem Leben, dem Universum und allem?"
> „Ja [...] die Antwort auf die Große Frage [...] lautet [...] Zweiundvierzig." [...]
> „Ist das alles, nach siebeneinhalb Millionen Jahren Denkarbeit?"
> „Ich habe es gründlich geprüft", sagte der Computer, „und das ist die Antwort, mit Sicherheit. Das Problem, wenn ich mal ganz ehrlich sein darf, scheint mir zu sein, dass ihr selbst nie gewusst habt, wie die Frage lautet."
> (Adams 2004: 49–50)

Diese prominente Szene von Douglas Adams Roman ‚Per Anhalter durch die Galaxis' verweist mit einer Prise Humor gleich auf zwei Umstände: Zum einen auf die Schwierigkeit, in Situationen von Sinnlosigkeit eine Antwort auf die Frage nach dem Sinn zu finden. Zweiundvierzig als Antwort ist für die Fragestellenden nur wenig hilfreich, mutet vielmehr sinnlos an. Zum anderen deutet der Computer *Deep Thought* an, dass die Probleme um Sinn bereits mit der Frage selbst und nicht erst mit der schwer zu findenden Antwort beginnen. Worin also liegt der Sinn der Sinnfrage?

Um genau dieser Frage näher zu kommen, werden wir auf den nächsten Seiten verschiedene Zugänge und Perspektiven mit den Mitteln der analytischen

Philosophie und der Psychoanalyse schaffen. Ein Anspruch liegt hierbei darin, in den teils recht theoretisch anmutenden Gedanken Verbindungslinien zur eigenen Lebenspraxis zu finden. Um mit Garrett Thomson zu sprechen: „An understanding of the meaning of life must have some practical implications for the way that we conduct our lives“ (Thomson 2003: 10).

Am Anfang unserer Beschäftigung mit dem Thema gilt es, begriffliche Klarheiten zu erlangen, indem die Sinn-Frage in zwei Fragen aufgeteilt wird: In die Fragen (1) ‚Was ist *der Sinn* von x?‘ und (2) ‚Was ist *Sinn?*‘. Diese Unterscheidung zwischen Sinn *sein* (2) und Sinn *haben* (1) ist deshalb wichtig, weil man, um nach dem Sinn von etwas zu fragen – wie in (1) – erst einmal die Bedeutung des Wortes (2) klären muss. Frage 1 setzt also in gewisser Weise bereits eine Antwort auf Frage 2 voraus. Nur Frage 2 zu beantworten, ohne Rücksicht darauf zu nehmen, wie das Wort ‚Sinn‘ in der Sprache gebraucht wird, scheint ebenso nur wenig sinnvoll (um gleich Ihr intuitives Verständnis des Themenkomplexes Sinn anzusprechen, werte Leserin und werter Leser). Entgegen der Auffassung einiger Autoren findet man hierbei gute Gründe dafür, die Fragen 1 und 2 nicht isoliert voneinander zu beantworten, sondern sensibel dafür zu sein, dass sie aufeinander verweisen. Deshalb werden wir im nächsten Abschnitt damit beginnen, uns der Frage nach dem Sinn des Lebens (als Frage aus dem Bereich 1) darüber zu nähern, wie sie in der Alltagssprache gebraucht wird und was hierbei mit Sinn (2) gemeint ist.

Sinn-Frage: Der Gebrauch in der Sprache, oder: Wann ist etwas sinnvoll?

Verschiedene Abhandlungen analytischer Philosophen zeigen, dass die Frage nach dem Sinn des Lebens nicht in allen Lesarten eine sinnvolle Frage und nur in bestimmten überhaupt beantwortbar ist. „Zunächst sind wir uns oft gar nicht sicher, was wir mit der Frage nach dem Sinn des Lebens zu erfahren suchen,“ schreibt etwa Nielsen (2000: 231). Er stellt fest, dass die Frage nach dem Sinn des Lebens nicht in klarer, festgelegter Weise gebraucht wird, dass jedoch aus der Unbestimmtheit im Gebrauch nicht folgt, dass diese Frage nicht eine wichtige Funktion erfüllt oder dass sie generell unbeantwortbar wäre. Die Frage weicht zwar nicht vom gewöhnlichen Sprachgebrauch ab, berührt aber ein tieferes Problem. Ihm zufolge will man bei der Frage wissen:

> Ist das Leben eine nichts sagende Sache nach der anderen, bis zu dem Tag, an dem wir sterben und zu verwesen beginnen? Oder kann ich es zusammenfassen und einen Witz darin

> finden? Oder ihm zumindest selbst einen Witz geben? Oder wäre das nur eine dumme Einbildung, geboren aus Angst und Zittern? (Nielsen 2000: 231)

In ihrer typischen Verwendungsweise fragt man dabei also nach den erstrebenswerten Zielen des Lebens oder auch, ob es im Leben überhaupt erstrebenswerte Ziele gebe. Eine unzulängliche Deutung wäre deshalb, wenn man die Frage nach dem Sinn des Lebens als eine *Tatsachenfrage* auffasst und fragt „Welche Funktion hat das Leben?" oder „Wozu wurde das Leben geschaffen?" in einem ähnlichen Sinn wie „Zu welchem Zweck betreibt man Gehirnchirurgie?" oder auch „Welche Funktion haben Regenschirme?" Bei derartigen Fragen ist man auf der Suche nach Erklärungen. Gibt man bei ihnen eine beliebige Antwort, zeigt man nur, wie etwas ist, aber man begründet nichts: „Selbst die vollständigste Erklärung oder Beschreibung davon, *wie* sich alles verhält, kann die ganz andere Frage nach dem Warum nicht beantworten" (Nielsen 2000: 233).

Näher an der Alltagsbedeutung ist man deshalb, wenn man die Frage nach dem Sinn des Lebens als *Wertfrage* auffasst und darin nach Begründungen fragt, im Sinne von: „Wie sollte man leben?" oder „Welche Lebensführung verdient mehr Wertschätzung als andere?" Bei diesen Fragen geht es einem darum, das zu erkennen, was wirklich wertvoll ist. Entscheidend ist, dass man aus Antworten auf Tatsachenfragen nicht auf Antworten auf Wertfragen schließen kann, d. h.: keine Tatsache kann für sich genommen eine Antwort auf die Sinnfrage als Wertfrage sein, kann beantworten, was wertvoll ist. Für sich genommen können weder (therapeutisch gewonnene) Einsichten in die eigene psychische Struktur noch religiöse Annahmen sinnstiftend sein, wenn man die Sinn-Frage als Wertfrage versteht.

Eine Ausnahme stellt allerdings die sog. *Grenzfrage* dar: Bei ihr wird die Sinnfrage dezidiert nicht als Wertfrage gestellt wird, sondern man sucht genau nach eben jenen genannten objektiven Tatsachen. Der Clou dabei ist, dass sich Tatsachen auch hier nicht als Antwort eignen, genau das jedoch gewollt ist. Wie ist das gemeint? Deutlich wird das, wenn man versteht, dass Grenzfragen zwar Fragen sind, „deren Form aus vertrauten Argumentationsformen übernommen wurde, die aber nicht die Funktion erfüllen, die sie innerhalb dieser Argumentationsformen gewöhnlich erfüllen" (Nielsen 2000: 234). Die Oberflächengrammatik einer Grenzfrage scheint zwar darauf hinzuweisen, dass es sich um eine vernünftige Frage handelt, aber ihre Tiefenstruktur zeigt, dass sie jenseits des Bereichs rationaler Äußerungen liegt. Die beiden Fragen „Worauf steht die Welt?" und „Worauf steht der Weihnachtsbaum?" sind der Form nach zwar sehr ähnliche Fragen, jedoch ist nur die zweite direkt beantwortbar; die erste eine Grenzfrage, bei der eine direkte Antwort die Person, die die Frage stellt, nicht zufriedenstellen kann und lediglich zur Wiederholung der Ausgangsfrage führen würde, bei der aber genau dies intendiert sein kann, etwa um eine persönliche Notlage auszudrücken. Beispiele hierfür wären der Ausruf „Warum ich?“ oder „Warum musste er leiden / sterben?“ Ansonsten handelt es sich dabei um einen Kategorienfehler im Sinne von „Wo ist irgendwo?“ oder „Was heißt blau?“.

Nielsens wichtige Analyse der Alltagssprache muss an dieser Stelle noch um die vielzitierte Position Wittgensteins ergänzt werden:

> Wir fühlen, daß selbst, wenn alle ‚möglichen‘ wissenschaftlichen Fragen beantwortet sind, unsere Lebensprobleme noch gar nicht berührt sind. Freilich bleibt dann eben keine Frage mehr; und eben dies ist die Antwort.
> Die Lösung des Problems des Lebens merkt man am Verschwinden dieses Problems.
> (Ist nicht dies der Grund, warum Menschen, denen der Sinn des Lebens nach langen Zweifeln klar wurde, warum diese dann nicht sagen konnten, worin dieser Sinn bestand.)
> (Wittgenstein 2001: Tractatus 6.52 und 6.521)

Ähnlich wie bei den Grenzfragen würde man Wittgenstein zufolge vergeblich nach einer konkreten Antwort auf das „Problem des Lebens“ suchen. Denn diese Frage entspringe einem gewissen Lebensvollzug (dies kann auch für die Sinn-Frage als Wertfrage gelten, auch wenn Wittgenstein dies nicht so sah) und zeige einem an, dass man sein Leben ändern solle. Gelänge es einem, sein Leben zu ändern, wäre das Problem der Frage gelöst – und das hieße bei ihm schlichtweg, die Frage verschwindet.

Die Betrachtung unserer Alltagssprache zeigt damit, dass wir, wenn wir die Sinn-Frage stellen, entweder auf eine Antwort darauf aus sind, was wertvoll ist und wie zu leben gut ist. Oder unsere gesuchte „Antwort“ ist überhaupt gar keine sprachliche, sondern wir wollen vielmehr unsere Not, unser Leiden ausdrücken und tragen damit auch den Wunsch der Beseitigung der Notlage durch eine Veränderung des Lebens an.

Sinn-Begriff: Abstecken des semantischen Feldes rund um ‚Sinn‘

Nach der Exploration der ganzen Frage nach dem Sinn – man kann sagen, der Sinnfrage in ihrer alltagssprachlichen ‚Gestalt‘ – verkleinern wir nun den Untersuchungsfokus mit dem Blick in die Semantik in Abb. 1 (Gomperz 1929, Lampersberger 2013, Thies 2008).

Eingedenk der vorangestellten Unterscheidung zwischen Sinn sein und Sinn haben kann dasjenige, das Sinn zur Fülle ‚hat‘, als ‚sinnvoll‘ definiert und von demjenigen abgegrenzt werden, das ‚sinnlos‘ ist, also keine Fülle ‚hat‘. Aufgrund der nicht vorhandenen Abstufungen in ‚sinnvoll‘ und ‚sinnlos‘ lässt sich zwischen

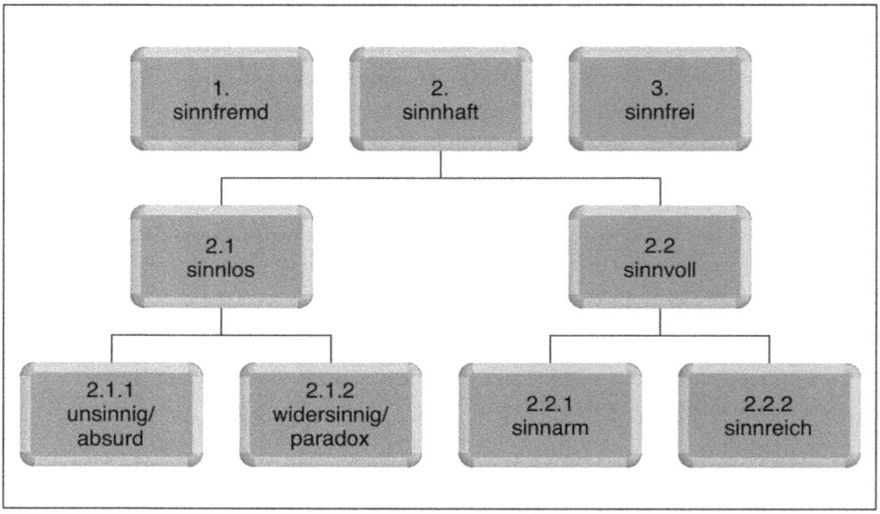

Abbildung 5.1 Semantisches Feld um den Sinn-Begriff (Lampersberger 2013: 76. Orientiert an Thies 2008)

mehr oder weniger Sinn im Bereich des ‚Sinnhaften' durch das Sprechen von ‚sinnarm' und ‚sinnreich' unterscheiden. Abgrenzen kann man das ‚Sinnhafte' vom ‚Sinnfremdem', welches nicht Träger von Sinn sein kann. Hier würde man sich eines Kategorienfehlers schuldig machen, wenn man den Sinnbegriff darauf anwenden würde (vgl. Grenzfrage). Bei dem ‚Sinnfreien' hingegen wird uns kein weiteres Verständnis zugemutet. Hier müssen wir schlichtweg nichts deuten, einordnen oder vorstellen, weil wir es gar nicht können. Die meisten derer, die dafür argumentieren, dass die Frage nach dem Sinn des Lebens falsch gestellt sei, weil das Leben als Sinnträger nicht in Frage komme, sprechen vom Leben als Sinnfremdem oder Sinnfreiem. ‚Unsinniges' oder auch ‚Absurdes' kennzeichnet etwas, das zwar prinzipiell sinnvoll sein kann, es aber in dem betrachteten Fall nicht ist, z. B. lexikalischer Unsinn in Form von Buchstabenfolgen ohne semantischen Sinn, oder auch Verhaltensweisen, die so ohne Weiteres nicht zu verstehen sind. Wenn Äußerungen und Handlungen zwar sinnvolle Elemente beinhalten, jedoch ein nicht sinnvolles Ganzes bilden, spricht man von etwas als ‚widersinnig', ‚sinnwidrig' oder ‚paradox'. Widersinniges lässt sich im Gegensatz zum Unsinnigen nicht zusammennehmen, nicht denken, wie etwa ein rundes Quadrat.

Eine kurze Bestandsaufnahme nach der dargestellten Differenzierung: Es gilt bisher, dass ein x nur dann mehr oder weniger Sinn haben kann (nicht Sinn *sein!*),

> wenn man sich mit dem x im Bereich des Sinn*haften* befindet, also die notwendigen Bedingungen erfüllt sind, dass x Träger von Sinn sein kann (nicht sinn*fremd*) und auch nicht inhaltslos ist (nicht sinn*frei*).

Für eine weitere wichtige Bedingung zum Gebrauch des Sinnbegriffs in der Sprache blicken wir kurz auf Robert Nozicks folgenden Hinweis: „Nach dem Sinn von etwas zu fragen heißt, wissen zu wollen, wie es mit anderen Dingen verknüpft ist" (Nozick 2002: 393). Sinn sieht er dadurch als gegeben an, dass wir bestimmte Grenzen transzendieren. Wir fügen damit hinzu: x kann Sinn haben,

> wenn man das x in ein anderes y, also in einen bestimmten Zusammenhang einordnen, integrieren kann.
>
> Dieses x verhält sich zu dem y wie ein „um willen"; y ist wesentlicher Teil der Antwort auf die Frage „Warum x?"

Letzteres findet sich u.a. in empirischen Forschungen zu Sinn als *Ultimate Meanings Technique* von Dmitry Leontiev (2007) und beim Forschungsteam von Tatjana Schnell als Interviewtechnik des „Leiterns" wieder:

> „Leitern" heißt, dass alle Antworten, die unsere Interviewpartner gaben, nochmals hinterfragt wurden: *Und warum? Wofür steht das für Sie? Was bedeutet das genau? Wofür steht das wiederum?* Diese Nachfragen wurden so oft wiederholt, bis eine grundlegende Bedeutung erreicht war, die nicht mehr hinterfragt werden konnte – bis wir also bei einer „Letztbedeutung" (*ultimate meaning, ultimate concern*, Lebensbedeutung) angekommen waren (Schnell 2016: 13).

Bis hierher können wir damit festhalten: Wenn man eine Antwort auf die Sinn-Frage geben möchte – insofern man die Antwort als sprachlich verfasst versteht und nicht als etwas ansieht, das durch eine bestimmte Art von Lebensvollzug gegeben wird, wie es im obigen Wittgenstein-Zitat anklingt – dann muss man davon ausgehen, dass Leben Träger von Sinn sein kann. Aber gehen wir, wie typisch für philosophische Analysen, erneut einen Schritt zurück und schauen uns noch einmal genauer an, was denn da eigentlich Sinn haben bzw. tragen soll. Ist dieses x wirklich das „Leben" und was hieße das genau?

Sinn-Träger: Was ist das Objekt der Sinnfrage und damit Träger von Sinn?

Bei der Klärung der Frage, was denn eigentlich Sinn haben soll, also was das Objekt der Sinn-Frage und damit der Träger von Sinn sein soll, ist es überaus hilfreich, verschiedene Ebenen voneinander zu unterscheiden. Denn während die Sinn-Frage zwar durchaus darauf abzielen kann, was sich allgemein wirklich lohnt, kann sie auch einen viel geringeren Radius haben, indem sie nach dem *Sinn einer bestimmten Handlung* fragt.[1] Die so Fragende will dabei wissen, wie sie in der Situation, in der sie eben ist, Sinn finden kann. Sie kann mit einem „Warum ist diese Handlung für mich sinnvoll?" (vgl. das „Leitern" oben) dann weiter fragen danach, ob dieser Sinn auch zu ihren übergeordneten Absichten oder gar zum Lebensplan passt. Bezeichnen wir dies mit Kauppinen (2012) als den *Sinn eines Lebensabschnitts*. Dieser wiederum müsste sich auf der nächsten Ebene des Verknüpftseins, der nächsten Integrationsebene (vgl. Nozick oben) in den jeweiligen Lebenssinn einfügen lassen. Hierbei ließen sich dazu passende Konzepte nennen, wie das von Harry Frankfurts (1988) grundsätzlichem „Caring" einer Person, oder Holmer Steinfaths (2001) Grundeinstellungen als fundamentalste Antwort, wie zu leben gut ist. Bis hierhin ist es (nach bestimmter, noch weiter unten zu bestimmender Lesart) möglich, derartige Fragen als Fragen nach dem Sinn *im* Leben zu verstehen (zur genaueren Unterscheidung vgl. Lampersberger 2014). Erweitert man die Perspektive über das einzelne Leben hinaus, so fragt man nach dem Sinn *des* jeweiligen Lebens. Dabei wird das beschriebene „um willen" von der einen Person, deren Sinn in Frage steht, auf andere Personen bzw. allgemein auf etwas über sie Hinausreichendes erweitert (z. B. einen größeren Zweck). So kann man etwa einen solchen Sinn des Lebens von Sigmund Freud darin sehen, dass er als Begründer der Psychoanalyse einen über seine Person hinausgehenden Diskurs über Unbewusstes eröffnete, der das Verständnis der menschlichen Psyche und die Behandlung psychisch Erkrankter voranbrachte. Auch hier muss man natürlich nicht stehenbleiben und könnte die Perspektive so lange erweitern, bis man gar zur ontologischen Frage nach dem *Sinn menschlichen Lebens allgemein* kommt. Schließlich kann dieser erfragte Sinn wieder in die grundlegende philosophische Frage des Sinns des Lebens allgemein münden, als Sinn des ganzen Kosmos, als die Leibniz'sche Frage „Warum gibt es überhaupt etwas und nicht vielmehr nichts?"

Doch wie hängen nun die Ebenen miteinander zusammen, vor allem die erste im Bereich des Sinnvollseins im jeweiligen Leben mit dem letzten Sinn des Lebens? Wird der Sinn einer einzelnen Handlung nur durch die Einordnung in einen globalen Sinn im jeweiligen gesamten Leben konstituiert oder gar erst durch den kosmischen Sinn? Setzt Sinn im Leben den viel größeren Sinn des Lebens voraus,

---

1 Man könnte – ginge es nicht lediglich um ein Aufzeigen einer groben möglichen Struktur – bei nachfolgender Einteilung natürlich noch viel kleinteiliger vorgehen und tief in verschiedene Mikroebenen gehen.

der alles andere begründet? Während Nozick genau dies meint, kann man mit Rückgriff auf die Reinhard Lauths (1953) Analyse verschiedene Momente des Sinnbegriffs dagegenhalten. Denn in seiner Habilitation argumentiert er, dass man bei der Eingliederung bzw. beim Transzendieren von Grenzen (er nennt es den „Umfang des Sinnbereichs“) genau so weit gehen muss, bis man in der übergeordneten Ebene auf etwas stößt, das nicht nur als Mittel für etwas Anderes ist, sondern durch sich selbst bzw. in sich selbst wertvoll ist: bis man einen *positiven Selbstwert* oder gar *Endwert* findet. Dies fügt sich gut in die oben durchgeführte alltagssprachliche Analyse der Sinnfrage als Wertfrage ein. Wenn etwas also in sich wertvoll ist – d. h. intrinsischen bzw. inhärenten Wert hat – dann ist es nicht notwendig, dass der Sinn erst durch die nächsthöhere Ebene garantiert wird. In welche Richtung diese Frage weist bzw. wie weit man beim „Leitern“ gehen muss, hängt damit davon ab, ob man das Wertvolle in der größeren oder in der kleineren Sache sieht. Selbstverständlich gibt es aber auch Selbstwerte, die zusätzlich noch Mittel für etwas anderes sind. Dies kann den Sinngehalt bzw. Sinnreichtum (s.o.) grundsätzlich noch erhöhen. Also etwa, wenn Freud sein Junktim aus Forschen und Heilen für sich allein als sinnvoll erlebt hat (Sinn im Leben für ihn) und die daraus entstandenen Erkenntnisse sinnvoll für über ihn Hinausgehendes sind (Sinn des Lebens für andere).

Sinn-Positionen: Konzepte in der philosophischen Debatte über Sinnkonzeptionen

Nach diesen basalen Untersuchungen blicken wir nun darauf, wie sich unsere Erkenntnisse in vollständigere Konzeptionen einfügen lassen, die ein wenig mehr Praxis in die Theorien bringen. Mithilfe von Thaddeus Metz (2001, 2002, 2013a) lassen sich grob drei Lager von am Wert ausgerichteten Sinntheorien in der philosophischen Debatte finden, die verschiedene Antworten darauf geben, wie man leben solle, um ein sinnvolles Leben zu führen.

Das erste Lager, der *Supernaturalismus*, beschreibt ein sinnvolles Leben als ein solches, welches einen Bezug zu etwas Höherem hat. Nach den *Gott-zentrierten supernaturalistischen* Theorien sorgt die Verbindung zu Gott für Sinn im Leben: Das eigene Leben sei umso sinnvoller, je mehr man den Zweck erfülle, den Gott für einen selbst bestimmt habe oder je mehr man die göttliche Natur ausdrücke, die in einem selbst angelegt sei. Die Grundidee besteht häufig darin, dass Gott so etwas wie einen Plan für das Universum habe und dass das eigene Leben in dem Grad sinnvoll sei, in dem man Gott dabei helfe, diesen Plan umzusetzen. Scheitert man darin, das zu leisten, was Gott mit seinem Leben geplant hat, so ist das eigene Leben sinnlos. Am prominentesten sind hier die sog. „Higher-Purpose-Theorien“, denen zufolge man von Gott für einen Zweck geschaffen sei, der den einzigen Weg darstelle, zu vermeiden, dass das eigene Leben kontingent sei. *Seelenzentrierte supernaturalistische* Theorien benötigen keine Existenz Gottes für Sinnerleben, verlangen allerdings, dass man seine „Seele“ (häufig ohne die notwendigen metaphysischen Überlegungen zu entwickeln) in einen bestimmten Zustand bringen muss, damit das eigene Leben sinnvoll sein kann.

Vertreter des *Naturalismus* hingegen gehen davon aus, dass selbst ohne „spiritual realm“ eine sinnvolle Existenz in einer rein physikalischen Welt möglich ist. Sowohl subjektive als auch objektive Varianten hiervon existieren. Nach dem *subjektiven Naturalismus* ist das, was für eine Person sinnvoll ist, abhängig von ihren personalen mentalen Zuständen, worunter insbesondere ihre Intentionen, Ziele, Projekte und Ideale fallen. Das Leben ist aus dieser Perspektive umso sinnvoller, je mehr man das bekommt, was einem selbst wichtig ist. Und das, was einem selbst wichtig ist, kann nicht von außen – d. h. personunabhängig – bestimmt werden, sondern nur in Bezug auf eine bestimmte Person in ihrem bestimmten Leben. Davon unabhängige Werte gäbe es nicht. Ein zentrales Problem solch rein subjektiver Theorien wird durch das Herausgreifen einer voluntaristischen Position offenkundig, wie der von Richard Taylor (2002). Er verändert den Mythos von Sisyphos in der Art, dass die Götter Sisyphos so unter Drogen setzen, dass jener – im Unterschied zu seinem drogenfreien Zustand – meint, es gäbe nichts Besseres und Sinnvolleres, als bis in alle Ewigkeiten Steine den Berg hochzutragen. Kritiker dieser Theorie (s. etwa unten Wolf) bemängeln, dass ein rein subjektives Sinnerleben nicht hinreichend für Sinn sein, wenn das Verwirklichte ganz offensichtlich nicht wertvoll ist. Mit Kauppinen gesprochen: „Just as a food can be unhealthy for a person even if she thinks it is healthy, a life can be meaningless for someone even if she thinks it is meaningful“ (Kauppinen 2012: 356).

Die *objektive* Variante des Naturalismus behauptet, dass zentrale Elemente des Sinns subjektunabhängig sind und mentale Zustände zur Sinn-Konstitution nicht hinreichen. Ein purer Objektivismus würde sogar so weit gehen, dass diese gar keine Rolle spielen. Die entscheidende Kritik setzt bei der Bestimmung der objektiven Werte an: Denn welche Werte gelten hier, warum tun sie dies und wer bestimmt das? Gängige Theorien diesbezüglich sind etwa Selbst-Transzendenz sowie Eingehen in organische Einheit und die Verwirklichung menschlicher Vollkommenheit. Aber auch das Ausdrücken nicht-hedonistischer Güter wie Freundschaft, Schönheit und Wissen findet sich oft, oder auch das der Verbesserung tierischen und menschlichen Lebens gewidmete Dasein.

Zuletzt sei nur kurz auf das dritte Lager hingewiesen, auf den *Nihilismus*, demzufolge es schlichtweg – Existenzialisten mögen dem Autor diese aus Platzgründen abgekürzte Überspitzung verzeihen – keinen Sinn gibt.

Eine Theorie, die in gewisser Weise ein Hybrid zwischen der subjektiven und objektiven Sicht darstellt und die bei vielen Sinn-Forschern Anklang findet, ist die Theorie von Susan Wolf. Nach Wolf (1998, 2010) besteht ein sinnerfülltes Leben darin, sich *aktiv mit lohnenswerten Projekten* und Vorhaben zu beschäftigen, wobei sie unter aktiver Beschäftigung versteht, dass ein Mensch von einer Sache ergriffen ist, diese ihn begeistert und berührt, sodass er sich ihr hingibt. In dieser Identifikation mit etwas sei man auf etwas Anderes als das eigene „Selbst" ausgerichtet. Wolf integriert damit die subjektive Seite, weil zu den Erfordernissen des Sinns auch die individuellen Sehnsüchte gehören, also das, was einem für das eigene Leben wirklich wichtig ist (s. etwa die Grundeinstellungen oben). Bestimmte Dinge berühren einen sehr tief und drücken dasjenige aus, was es für einen bedeutet, man selbst zu sein und gut zu leben. Eine lediglich objektive Theorie des Sinns würde akzeptieren, dass die Person von ihrem Sinn gelangweilt ist, dass er ihr nicht wichtig ist oder sie ihm gar entfremdet ist. Wolf betont jedoch mehrfach, dass es nicht um ein bloßes Erkennen oder Ausbilden einer Pro-Einstellung für das je Wichtige geht, sondern dass man für Sinnerleben eine aktive Beziehung zu dem Gegenstand einnehmen muss. Bereits das Hervorheben, dass man seine Projekte für erfüllend halten möchte, bereitet wiederum den Weg für die objektive(re) Seite, denn man will – so Wolf – nur von etwas erfüllt sein, dem etwas unbedingt Lohnenswertes oder Gutes anhaftet (und nicht wie Taylors Sisyphos, s.o.).

> [Es ist notwendig], daß die Idee der Sinnhaltigkeit ohne eine Unterscheidung zwischen lohnenswerten und weniger lohnenswerten Arten und Weisen, seine Zeit zu verbringen, keinen Sinn macht, wobei der Test, was lohnenswert ist, zumindest teilweise unabhängig von den unbegründeten Präferenzen oder Glücksempfinden eines Menschen sein soll (Wolf, 1998: 171).

Während es mit Wolfs Theorie durch ihre Verbindung von subjektiven und objektiven Elementen zwar gut gelingt, eine lebensnahe Sinn-Konzeption vorzustellen, so bleibt dennoch ein Problem bestehen, das vor allem in Krisenmomenten (und diese sind es ja häufig, die ein Sinnlosigkeitsgefühl mit sich bringen) virulent wird. Denn was ist, wenn es einer Person nicht (mehr) gelingt, sich aktiv mit erfüllenden Projekten zu beschäftigen, weil sie sowohl in ihrer inneren als auch der äußeren Welt nichts mehr als lohnenswert erleben kann? Was ist, wenn gewisse Voraussetzungen bzw. Fähigkeiten zum Suchen, Finden, Schaffen, Wahrnehmen, Gestalten und Erleben von Sinn nicht gegeben sind? Kann dies jeder Mensch oder gibt es manche, denen hierbei Schwierigkeiten in die Wiege gelegt sind? Und wie hängen Sinn und Krankheit bzw. Pathologie zusammen? Um diese Fragen zu beantworten und vor allem das *Erleben* von Sinnlosigkeit besser zu verstehen, müssen wir über die Philosophie hinausgehen, in den Bereich der Psychologie, Psychotherapie und v. a.: in die Psychoanalyse. Lange hat sich die Psychologie und Psychotherapie höchstens indirekt mit dem Thema Sinn beschäftigt (Metz 2013b), was bestimmt auch an Freud selbst lag, der 1937 in einem Brief an Marie Bonaparte schrieb:

> Im Moment, da man nach dem Sinn und Wert des Lebens fragt, ist man krank, denn beides gibt es ja in objektiver Weise nicht; man hat nur eingestanden, dass man einen Vorrat an unbefriedigter Libido hat, und irgend etwas anderes muss damit vorgefallen sein, eine Art Gärung, die zur Trauer und Depression führt (Freud 1960: 452).

Erst in den letzten Jahren kann ein steigendes Interesse der Psychotherapie an der Sinnfrage verzeichnet werden, wenn auch noch viel zu selten auf die philosophische Sinn-Debatte Bezug genommen wird.

Sinn-Fähigkeit: Hinreichend gute Objektbeziehung für sinnhaften Lebensvollzug

Um sich den eben gestellten Fragen zu nähern, blicken wir mittels der psychoanalytischen Objektbeziehungstheorie[2] auf gelingendes und misslingendes Ausbilden der Sinn-Fähigkeit. Mit Herbert Will (2005) gesprochen:

> Die Fähigkeit, Sinn zu erleben, entsteht in der Objektbeziehung. Das Baby erlebt unentwegt Situationen, Körperwahrnehmungen und Sensationen, die es nicht verstehen kann und von denen es überwältigt wird. Es braucht Personen, die ihm seine Welt erschließen helfen (Will 2005: 542).

Will weist auf folgende essentielle Bedingungen zum Sinn-Erleben hin, die im Weiteren näher ausgeführt werden: Die Fähigkeiten zu Symbolisierung, Mentalisierung und Besetzung.

---

2 Unter (äußerem) Objekt kann man sehr vereinfacht gesagt das Gegenüber verstehen, wie es v. a. in frühen Beziehungserfahrungen zu den primären Bindungspersonen verinnerlicht wird (und durch diese Internalisierung zum inneren Objekt wird). Vgl. etwa Schriften der zitierten Autoren Bion und Winnicott.

Grundlage für die Entwicklung all jener genannten Fähigkeiten, v. a. der basalen *Symbolisierungsfähikeit*, ist, dass die („good enough“) Bindungspersonen mit und für das Kind eine wohlwollende, als sicher erlebbare Atmosphäre („holding environment“) etablieren können, in dem sie ihm ihre affektive Regulierungsfunktion zur Verfügung stellen (Winnicott 1958). Dies bildet den stark verkürzten Hintergrund für einen für Sinn-Erleben notwendigen Prozess, den Wilfred Bion (1962b) als *Containing* bezeichnet hat. Dabei nimmt die Bezugsperson die unverarbeiteten und noch kaum symbolisierungsfähigen rohen mentalen Zustände (die sog. „Beta-Elemente“) – sei es ein unspezifisches Gefühl von Hunger oder etwa ein diffuses Gefühl von Angst – in sich auf. Auf das Kind eingestimmt („träumerisch denkend“ oder in „Reverie“, in der Sprache von Bion), macht sich die Bezugsperson dann ein Bild von den Gedanken und Gefühlen des Kindes und verarbeitet diese zunächst für sich, lässt sich darauf ein und stellt intra- und interpsychischen Raum dafür zur Verfügung, sie *contains*, ist der Container für die rohen Beta-Elemente des Kindes und „verdaut“ diese. Bion bezeichnet dies als die „Alpha-Funktion“. In einem nächsten Schritt gibt sie dem Kind die Zustände in erträglicher, verdauter Form zurück. Auf die Angst des Kindes reagiert sie also nicht gleich mit Angst oder gibt dem Kind die Angst unverdaut zurück. Das Kind kann dann dieses erträglichere Bild, aber auch die Alpha-Funktion internalisieren und dadurch Schritt für Schritt die Fähigkeit erlernen, Erlebnisse psychisch zu verarbeiten und als emotionale Erfahrungen zu integrieren. Die rohen Daten werden dadurch zu psychischen Inhalten, die Bedeutung haben können und zum Denken verwendet werden können. Gelingt dieser Vorgang nicht, so bleibt das Kind mit den für sich kaum einordenbaren und nicht symbolisierten Beta-Elementen zurück. Bion prägt hier den Begriff der nicht mit Bedeutung versehenen „namenlosen Angst“:

> Normal development follows if the relationship between infant and breast permits the infant to project a feeling, say, that it is dying into the mother and to reintroject it after its sojourn in the breast has made it tolerable to the infant psyche. If the projection is not accepted by the mother the infant feels that its feeling that it is dying is stripped of such meaning that it has. It therefore reintrojects, not a fear of dying made tolerable, but a nameless dread (Bion 1962a: 309).

Es liegt auf der Hand, wie basal wichtig die Alpha-Funktion für Sinnerleben ist und inwiefern bei traumatischen Erlebnissen und Erfahrungen von unsagbarem, nicht repräsentierbaren Leid nur wenig Möglichkeiten bestehen, aus dem Erlebten Sinn zu machen. Man verbleibt bis dahin im Bereich des Sinn-Fremden. Denn man muss Erlebtes erst einmal symbolisieren können, um mental damit agieren zu können – schlichtweg auch, um darüber nachdenken zu können, ohne komplett überwältigt zu sein – um sich Gedanken über die verschiedenen „Warums" und Verknüpfungsebenen von Sinn machen zu können.

Auch die *Mentalisierungsfähigkeit* als die „Fähigkeit, das eigene Verhalten sowie die Handlungsweisen anderer Menschen plausibel als Resultat zugrunde liegender psychischer Zustände zu interpretieren" (Bateman & Fonagy 2008: 128), nimmt eine basale (und eng mit der Symbolisierungsfähigkeit verschränkte) Rolle im Sinnerleben ein, weil nur qua dieser Ich-Funktion Sinn zugeschrieben werden und die Welt mit Bedeutung angereichert werden kann: „Mentalisierung erschafft die Welt als eine sinnreiche, und sie ermöglicht es wiederum erst, den Sinnreichtum zu erleben" (Will 2005: 547–548). Der psychische Umgang mit einer als bedeutsam erlebbaren Welt, bei dem nur künstlich zwischen Sinn-Erleben und Sinn-Herstellen unterschieden werden kann, geschieht vor dem Hintergrund verfügbarer Objektbeziehungen bzw. „geronnener Beziehungserfahrungen" (Luborsky & Crits-Christoph 1990). Man mag gar so weit gehen, dass diese Vorgänge im „Zwischen" von Innen und Außen geschehen, wie Winnicotts es in seinem Verständnis des Übergangsraums nahelegt: „It is in the space between inner and outer world, which is also the space between people – the transitional space – that intimate relationships and creativity occur" (Winnicott 1953: 92). Es ist dies der benötigte Raum für die Integration eines x in ein y (s. o.) und damit etwas für einen Wichtigkeit erlangen kann, oder in der Sprache Freuds: damit etwas *libidinös besetzt* werden kann. Letzteres ist ebenso notwendig für die Sinnfrage, die wir ja als Wertfrage verstanden wissen wollen. Gerade in der Depression ist diese Besetzung allerdings schwer, wird die Libido manchmal komplett von der Objektwelt abgezogen. Oder literarischer formuliert: „Bei Trauer ist die Welt arm und leer geworden, bei Melancholie ist es das Ich selbst" (Freud 1916-17 g: 431). Im Ich gibt es dann kaum mehr etwas, das als wertvoll erlebt werden kann, das Selbst und ausgehend davon die erlebte Welt wird grau, wird als sinnlos erlebt.

Sinn-Unbewusstes: Der verborgene, aber erschließbare Sinn psychischer Phänomene

Neben der Fähigkeit zum Sinn-Erleben vermag ein psychoanalytischer Blick noch Weiteres zum Sinn-Thema beizutragen, v. a. durch die für Psychoanalytikerinnen und Psychoanalytiker typische Offenheit dafür, dass hinter zunächst unverständlich erscheinenden psychischen Produkten ein verborgener (oft unbewusster) Sinn liegen könnte. So gilt im allgemeinen psychoanalytischen Störungsmodell (v. a. das neurotische) Symptom nicht als sinn-frei oder sinn-fremd, selbst wenn uns das Unbewusste häufig Un-Sinn oder gar zunächst Sinn-Widriges (s. Abschnitt 2) aufgibt:

> Als Antwort auf die innerseelische Konfliktverarbeitung reagiert der psychische Apparat mit der Bildung des neurotischen Symptoms. Der psychoanalytischen Vorstellung zufolge hat das neurotische Symptom einen Sinn, indem es auf den Konflikt verweist bzw. diesen symbolisiert (Jungclaussen 2013: 142).

Symptome können sich z. B. als Ergebnis einer Kompromissleistung zwischen andrängendem Wunsch und seiner Abwehr entpuppen. So kann man eine Armlähmung (Konversion) als Kompromiss zwischen dem Wunsch, zuzuschlagen (Aggression), und seiner Abwehr (durch Erschlaffung des Arms) verstehen. Die verschiedenen Abwehrbewegungen des Individuums, die unlösbar erscheinende Konflikte in das Unbewusste verschieben und dort halten, verfremden in diesen Fällen potentiellen Sinn. Umso neurotisch übersteigerter die Abwehr dabei ist, desto mehr wird das Herstellen und Erleben von sinnhaften Zusammenhängen erschwert, wenn nicht gar verunmöglicht – etwas, das umso mehr für primitive Abwehrmechanismen gilt (vgl. fehlende Alpha-Funktion oben bei Bion). Dies soll jedoch nicht darüber hinwegtäuschen, dass der angesprochene vermeintliche Un-Sinn auch Sinn-Potenzial mit sich bringen kann, da er eine nicht zu vernachlässigende Ich-Leistung darstellt:

> [Das Symptom ist] Ausdruck der Versuche des Subjekts, mit den Zwistigkeiten, Ungereimtheiten und Widersprüchen im eigenen Inneren zurechtzukommen und psychischen Schmerz in Grenzen zu halten. [...] Ob diese Ersatzbildungen nach außen als Verrücktheit, Neurose oder kreative Leistung mit künstlerischem „Wert" imponieren – immer sind sie eine kreative Schöpfung, eine Kreation des Subjekts (Müller-Pozzi 2008:211).

Die Betonung des Kreativen bei Müller-Pozzi, wie auch bereits zuvor bei Winnicotts Übergangsraum, lässt sich dabei auch als *Aufforderung zum Sinn* verstehen. So ist Viktor Frankl und vielen kontemporären Vertretern der Logotherapie und Existenzanalyse zu widersprechen, wenn sie dem „Willen zum Trieb" – welchen Frankl (2016) der Psychoanalyse unterstellte – den ihres Erachtens menschlicheren und eigentlicheren „Willen zum Sinn" entgegensetzen. Denn, so können wir nach unserer Abhandlung argumentieren, selbst das individuelle Triebleben einschließlich seiner unbewussten Tendenzen – ja das ganze Unbewusste – vermag zu einer sinnreicheren Gestaltung des Lebens aufzurufen:

> Insofern kann das Unbewusste sowohl – durch Ängste, Schuld- und Schamgefühle – signalisieren, dass dieses lebenswerte Leben noch nicht realisiert wurde; es kann aber auch durch Gefühle der Zufriedenheit, des Wohlbefindens oder des Glücks die Einsicht vermitteln, dass ein spezifischer Sinn verwirklicht wurde (Gödde & Zirfas 2016: 547).

Mit einem derartigen psychoanalytischen Verständnis ist bereits ein weiter Weg seit Freuds Brief von 1937 geschritten, der auch eine Versöhnung der noch stark voneinander abgewandten Lager Psychoanalyse und Logotherapie mit sich zu bringen vermag. Denn wenn wir qua Ernstnehmen des Unbewussten etwa aus dem Leben nach dem falschen Selbst herausfinden, uns hinter die Abwehr der emotionalen Versorgungswünsche bewegen können, im depressiven Einbruch erkennen, dass wir uns selbst in altruistischer Hilfsabtretung nicht mehr übersehen wollen, besteht die Möglichkeit zur Verwirklichung eines freieren und sinnreicheren Lebens. Sinn ist also nicht nur Thema sinnzentrierter Psychotherapien, sondern spielt mittlerweile in jeder Psychotherapie eine basale Rolle. Um abschließend mit Martin Altmeyer zu sprechen, der in folgendem Zitat die moderne Psychoanalyse seit Mitchell verortet:

> Der Patient brauche heute weniger das, was ihm die klassische Psychoanalyse angeboten bzw. abverlangt habe, also Aufklärung über die eigene Triebwelt, Verzicht auf infantile Wunschbefriedigungen, Anpassung an soziokulturelle Anforderungen, und erwarte vielmehr Unterstützung bei seiner individuellen Suche nach dem Sinn des Lebens, nach Authentizität und Vielfalt, nach persönlicher Identität ohne Identitätszwang. Der Analytiker wiederum besitze weder objektives noch exklusives Wissen über die Psyche seines Patienten; statt nach biografischer Wahrheit suche er gemeinsam mit dem Patienten nach den Bedeutungen, die in dessen Interaktionsgeschichte und Beziehungserfahrungen verborgen sind, einschließlich der Bedeutung der analytischen Beziehung selbst, und nach neuen Lebensentwürfen (Altmeyer 2011: 124).

Literatur

Adams D (2004) Das Leben, das Universum und alles. In: Fehige C et al. (Hg.) Sinn des Lebens. München: dtv. 43–52.

Altmeyer M (2011) Soziales Netzwerk Psyche – Versuch einer Standortbestimmung der modernen Psychoanalyse. Forum Psychoanalyse 27:107–127.

Bateman AW, Fonagy P (2008) Psychotherapie der Borderline Persönlichkeitsstörung. Ein mentalisierungsgestütztes Behandlungskonzept. Gießen: Psychosozialverlag.

Bion WR (1962a) A Theory of Thinking. In Spillius EB (Hg.) Melanie Klein Today: Developments in theory and practice. London: Routledge. 306–310.

Bion WR (1962b) Learning from experience. London: Tavistock.

Frankfurt HG (1988) The importance of what we care about: Philosophical essays. New York: Cambridge University Press.

Frankl VE (2016) Der Wille zum Sinn. Bern: Hogrefe.

Freud S (1916–17 g) Trauer und Melancholie, GW X: 428–446.

Freud S (1960) Briefe aus dem Jahr 1937. An Marie Bonaparte. In Freud EL & Freud L (Hg.) Briefe 1873–1939. Frankfurt a. M.: S. Fischer. 452.

Gomperz H (1929) Über Sinn und Sinngebilde – Verstehen und Erklären. Tübingen: Siebeck.

Gödde G, Zirfas J (2016) Therapeutik und Lebenskunst. Gießen: Psychosozial-Verlag.

Jungclaussen I (2013) Handbuch Psychotherapie-Antrag. Psychodynamisches Verständnis und effizientes Berichtschreiben in der tiefenpsychologisch fundierten Psychotherapie. Stuttgart: Schattauer.
Kauppinen A (2012) Meaningfulness and Time. Philosophy and Phenomenological Research 84(2):345 – 377.
Lampersberger F (2013) Sinn – philosophisch. Spiritual Care 2(1):76 – 79.
Lampersberger F (2014) Eine philosophische Untersuchung des Sinnbegriffs: In Logotherapie und Existenzanalyse von Viktor Frankl. Saarbrücken: AV Akademikerverlag.
Lauth R (1953) Die Frage nach dem Sinn des Daseins. Ausgabe 2002, München: Jerrentrup.
Leontiev DA (2007) Approaching worldview structure with ultimate meanings technique. Journal of Humanistic Psychology 47(2):243 – 266.
Luborsky L, Crits-Christoph P (1990) Understanding Transference. New York: Basic Books.
Metz T (2001) The Concept of a Meaningful Life. In: American Philosophical Quarterly 38(2):137 – 153.
Metz T (2002) Recent Work on the Meaning of Life. Ethics 112 (4):781 – 814.
Metz T (2013a) Meaning in Life. An Analytic Study. New York: Oxford University Press.
Metz T (2013b) Meaning in Life as the Aim of Psychotherapy: A Hypothesis. In: Hicks JA & Routledge C (Hg.) The Experience of Meaning in Life: Clasical Perspectives, Emerging Themes and Controversies. Dordrecht: Springer. 405 – 417.
Müller-Pozzi H (2008) Eine Triebtheorie für unsere Zeit – Sexualität und Konflikt in der Psychoanalyse. Bern: Huber.
Nielsen K (2000) Analytische Philosophie und der „Sinn des Lebens“. In: Fehige C et al. (Hg.) Sinn des Lebens. München: dtv. 228 – 251.
Nozick R (2002) In: Fehige C et al. (Hg.) Sinn des Lebens. München: dtv. 377 – 407.
Schnell T (2016) Psychologe des Lebenssinns. Berlin Heidelberg: Springer.
Steinfath H (2001) Orientierung am Guten: praktisches Überlegen und die Konstitution von Personen. Frankfurt a. M.: Suhrkamp.
Taylor R (2002) Sisyphos und wir. In: Fehige C et al. (Hg.) Sinn des Lebens. München: dtv. 87 – 495.
Thies C (2008) Der Sinn der Sinnfrage – Metaphysische Reflexionen auf kantianischer Grundlage. München: Herder.
Thomson G (2003) On the meaning of life. South Melbourne: Wadsworth.
Will H (2005) Über die Fähigkeit, Sinn zu schaffen und Sinn zu erleben. Eine psychoanalytische Skizze. In Petzold H & Orth I (Hg.) Sinn, Sinnerfahrung, Lebenssinn in Psychologie und Psychotherapie. Bielefeld: Aisthesis. 535 – 560.
Winnicott D (1953) Transitional objects and transitional phenomena. International Journal of Psycho-Analysis 34:89 – 97.
Winnicott D (1958) The capacity to be alone. International Journal of Psycho-Analysis 39:416 – 420.
Wittgenstein L (2001) Tractatus logico-philosophicus. Berlin: Akademie-Verlag.

Johannes Nathschläger

Zwischen Sinn und Dystopie

Der „Wille zum Sinn“ und die Vision des „Homo Deus“

Between meaning and dystopia: the „will to meaning“ and the vision of „homo deus“

Zusammenfassung: In diesem Beitrag wird der von Viktor E. Frankl (1905 – 1997) proklamierte „Wille zum Sinn“ als primäre Motivationskraft des Menschen mit dem dystopisch anmutenden Szenario eines technologischen und medizinischen Fortschrittes konfrontiert, durch welchen sich der Mensch im 21. Jahrhundert schrittweise selbst vergöttlicht. Diese Position, vertreten durch den israelischen Historiker Yuval N. Harari (*1976), fordert die anthropologischen Paradigmen heraus, welche Frankl Mitte des 20. Jahrhunderts formulierte und die wegweisend für die von ihm begründete Logotherapie als sinnzentrierte Psychotherapie wurden. In diesem Artikel soll daher insbesondere der Frage nachgegangen werden, wie der Mensch unter den genannten Vorzeichen im 21. Jahrhundert noch Sinn finden kann – und, nicht zuletzt, ob wir es dabei künftig überhaupt noch mit jenem Menschen zu tun haben, der von Frankl im Kern als „geistige Person“ begriffen wurde.

Schlüsselwörter: Dataismus, Digitalisierung, Existenzielles Vakuum, Frankl, Geist, geistige Person, Harari, Homo Deus, Logotherapie, Sinn, Sinnverwirklichung

Abstract: In this article, the “will to meaning” proclaimed by Viktor E. Frankl (1905 – 1997) as the primary motivational force of human beings is confronted with the apparently dystopian scenario of technological and medical progress through which humans in the 21st Century have gradually deified themselves. This position, represented by the Israeli historian Yuval N. Harari, challenges the anthropological paradigms which Frankl formulated in the mid-20th century and which pioneered the logotherapy he founded as meaning-centered psychotherapy. This article will therefore deal in particular with the question of how humans can still find meaning under the aforementioned signs in the 21st century – and, not least, whether we will still be dealing with the same human being that Frankl essentially understood as a “spiritual person”.

https://doi.org/10.1515/9783110787153-006

Keywords: dataism, digitalization, existential vacuum, Frankl, spirit, spiritual person, Harari, Homo Deus, logotherapy, meaning, realization of meaning

Einleitung

Wenn man sich im gegenwärtigen logotherapeutischen Diskurs umsieht, dann richtet sich dort immer wieder der Blick auf die Frage, welche Zukunft dieser sogenannten „3. Wiener Schule der Psychotherapie" (nach der Psychoanalyse Sigmund Freuds und der Individualpsychologie Alfred Adlers) beschieden sei. Als sinn- und wertorientierte Form der Psychotherapie könne die Logotherapie in unruhigen und unsicheren Zeiten jene Orientierung bieten, welche den Menschen von heute genauso ansprechen könne wie in der Mitte des 20. Jahrhunderts, als Viktor Frankl viele seiner grundlegenden Schriften veröffentlichte (Vgl. insbesondere Frankl 1955, Frankl 1972, Frankl 1975 und Frankl 1978).

Als ein Beispiel, auf welches im Sinne einer Parallelität immer wieder gerne Bezug genommen wird, soll hier Frankls Argumentation für eine *Pathologie des Zeitgeistes* (vgl. Biller & de Lourdes Stiegeler 2017: 281–287) genannt werden. Damit meinte Frankl die Fähigkeit des Menschen, kraft seiner geistigen Person den jeweiligen Umständen auf körperlicher oder psychischer Ebene entgegentreten zu können, mithin ihnen zu trotzen (vgl. Frankl 1985/1998: 63–66). Damit argumentiert Frankl gegen reduktionistische Menschenbilder, die den Einzelnen durch seine biologischen und sozialen Umstände determiniert sehen.

Doch hält die Lehre Frankls auch den gravierenden Veränderungen stand, die uns als Menschheit im Zuge dessen bevorstehen, was im Allgemeinen unter dem Namen *Digitalisierung* oder auch *digitale Revolution* (vgl. hierzu Brynjolfsson & McAfee 2019) beschrieben wird? Und wie verändert sich unser Leben hier beispielsweise durch den medizinischen und biotechnologischen Fortschritt? Kurzum: Bleibt der Mensch angesichts der in verschiedenen Szenarien prognostizierten Veränderungen in seiner Sinnorientiertheit unberührt? Oder verändert sich unser Leben so grundlegend, dass wir es in naher Zukunft mit einer posthumanen Spezies zu tun bekommen, die sich selbst durch technologischen Fortschritt soweit optimiert hat, dass sie strenggenommen (von äußeren Ähnlichkeiten abgesehen) nicht mehr viel mit dem menschlichen Leben zu tun hat, das uns heute noch vertraut ist?

Um diese und damit zusammenhängende Fragen zu diskutieren und möglichen Antworten zuzuführen, sollen daher zunächst kurz Frankls Hauptwege zur Sinnverwirklichung dargestellt werden, die gleichsam eine Kernüberzeugung seiner Lehre zum Ausdruck bringen (1). Im nächsten Schritt soll dann kritisch gefragt werden, ob sich diese Sinnmöglichkeiten im weiteren Fortgang des

21. Jahrhunderts im Zuge des digitalen und medizinischen Fortschrittes überhaupt noch weiter verwirklichen lassen werden – oder ob sich der Mensch gerade durch den Fortschritt paradoxerweise seiner Sinnmöglichkeiten im Begriff ist zu berauben (2). Um genau diese Bedenken inhaltlich zuzuspitzen, wird dann die Position des israelischen Historikers Yuval N. Harari hinzugezogen, der den Menschen auf dem Weg hin zu einem *Homo Deus* (Harari 2019) sieht, der sich immer weiter von dem entkoppelt, was unsere Lebensform bislang ausgemacht hat (3). Abschließend sollen die Überlegungen in drei Antwortversuchen münden – Antworten aus logotherapeutischer Perspektive auf Fragen, die Harari am Ende von *Homo Deus* zur Diskussion stellt (4).

Frankls drei Wege zur Sinnverwirklichung durch Wertverwirklichung

Gemäß Viktor Frankl findet der Mensch Sinn durch die Verwirklichung von Werten (vgl. Frankl 1946/2017: 91–95). Hierfür benennt er drei Wertkategorien: Schöpfungswerte, Erlebniswerte und Einstellungswerte. Bei den *Schöpfungswerten* geht es, vereinfacht gesagt, um die Verwirklichung von Werten, die auf einer Tätigkeit bzw. einem Handeln des Menschen beruhen. *Sinn* wird hier verwirklicht durch ein selbsttranszendentes Wirken, also ein Wirken auf einen Wert, der jenseits meiner selbst liegt. Dies geschieht hauptsächlich durch (sinnvolle) Arbeit, ehrenamtliche Tätigkeiten, aber auch durch die Kunst, beispielsweise durch Malerei oder Musik. Alle diese schöpferischen Tätigkeiten werden durchgeführt, um einen Wert zu verwirklichen, der außerhalb meiner selbst liegt – z. B. zum Wohle der Gemeinschaft, der Familie, des Unternehmens, des Betrachters oder Zuhörers usw. Natürlich ist nicht jede Tätigkeit schöpferisch und sinnvoll, insbesondere auch unter ethischen Gesichtspunkten. Als Seismograph bezüglich der Sinnhaftigkeit kann uns laut Frankl das Gewissen als eine Art „Sinn-Organ“ dienen (Frankl 1946/2017: 87).

Die zweite Kategorie stellen bei Frankl die *Erlebniswerte* dar. Gemeint ist damit zweierlei (vgl. Frankl 1981/1997b: 61). Zum einen geht es um die *Liebe* im Sinne einer wiederum selbsttranszendenten Tätigkeit – ein *über-sich-selbst-hinaus* und *auf jemanden-anderes-hin*. In der Liebe lassen wir uns ganz und gar auf einen anderen Menschen ein. Das Wesen der Liebe ist deshalb ebenso selbsttranszendent wie eine schöpferische Tätigkeit. In dem wir ganz und gar von uns selbst absehen und uns jemand anderen liebend hingeben, verwirklichen wir Sinn und erfahren Sinnhaftigkeit. Zum anderen geht es bei der Verwirklichung von Erlebniswerten auch noch um etwas Allgemeineres, nämlich Sinnverwirklichung durch Erlebniswerte. Nicht nur in der schöpferischen Tätigkeit der Kunst, sondern auch im Kunstgenuss kann der Mensch Sinn erfahren. Auch im Sammeln von Erfahrung, beispielsweise durch Reisen und dem Kennenlernen neuer Menschen und Kulturen können Erlebniswerte verwirklicht werden. Denn auch hier kommt das transzendente Wesen des Menschen zum Tragen – in Form der Aufmerksamkeitsverschiebung weg von mir selbst, auf etwas oder jemand anderen hin.

Als dritte Wertkategorie nennt Frankl die *Einstellungswerte*. Sie kommen einerseits vor allem überall dort zum Tragen, wo die Verwirklichung von anderen Schöpfungs- und Erlebniswerten nicht oder nicht mehr möglich ist. Andererseits aber auch dort, wo sich der einzelne Mensch mit schicksalhaftem, unabänderlichem Leid konfrontiert sieht, welches sich nicht mehr ändern, jedoch zumindest noch gestalten lässt – und zwar vor allem durch die *Haltung* die man dazu einnimmt. So kann beispielsweise ein unheilbar an Krebs erkrankter Patient durch eine innere Haltung der Tapferkeit und Zuversicht seinen Mitmenschen Vorbild sein und den mit-leidenden Angehörigen Trost spenden. So wird auch bei der Verwirklichung von Einstellungswerten wiederum ein selbsttranszendentes Moment erkennbar.

Man kann also festhalten: Sinnverwirklichung geschieht für Frankl durch Wertverwirklichung – und diese geschieht wiederum grob auf den drei skizzierten Wegen. Gemeinsam ist den unterschiedlichen Wegen der selbsttranszendente Charakter. Erst durch unsere Abwendung von uns selbst und unsere Hinwendung auf anderes hin lässt sich Sinn verwirklichen.

Wenn Menschen nun einen Mangel an Sinn empfinden, dann kann dies zum Zustand des *Existenziellen Vakuums* führen, der potentiell pathologisch werden kann, insbesondere wenn dieser Mangel an Sinn im eigenen Leben über einen längeren Zeitraum hinweg erfahren wird. Frankl prägte dafür den Begriff der *noogenen Neurose*, einer Störung also, die im Geistigen (altgr. *Nous*) liegt, wobei in Frankls dreidimensionalem Menschenbild nur die Dimensionen des Körpers und der Psyche erkranken können, nicht aber der Geist (vgl. Frankl 1981/1997b: 114). Durch die geistige Dimension ist es uns erst möglich, Werte und Wertmöglichkeiten wahrzunehmen, Sinn zu verwirklichen bzw. unter Sinnlosigkeit zu leiden.

Sinnverwirklichung im 21. Jahrhundert: Herausforderungen und Gefahren

Jeder technologische Fortschritt bringt auch die Notwendigkeit einer Antwort auf mögliche unerwünschte Nebenwirkungen mit sich. Oder, im Geiste der Postmoderne ausgedrückt: Fortschritte sind nie eindeutig, sondern potentiell immer mehrdeutig und durchzogen von Ambivalenzen und Paradoxien (vgl. Lyotard 1979). Unter der Zielstellung des Artikels soll sich der Blick im Weiteren nun auf einige dieser Ambivalenzen und Paradoxien richten. Für alle drei von Frankl beschriebenen Wertkategorien lassen sich solche aufzeigen.

Schöpfungswerte: Die Veränderungen auf dem Arbeitsmarkt durch die fortschreitende digitale Revolution sind bereits seit einigen Jahren Bestandteil des politischen und öffentlichen Diskurses. Unter dem Namen „Arbeitswelt 4.0" geht es dabei u. a. um die Flexibilisierung von Arbeitsorten und -zeiten bei gleichzeitigem Schutz von Arbeitnehmerrechten (vgl. hierzu Fortmann & Kolocek 2019). Darüber hinaus wendet sich der Blick aber auch zunehmend auf Szenarien, die davon ausgehen, dass in Zukunft viele Arbeitsplätze durch Automatisierung und Digitalisierung wegfallen und Millionen von heute noch beschäftigten Arbeitnehmerinnen und Arbeitnehmern künftig nicht mehr gebraucht werden (vgl. Precht 2018). In die gleiche Kerbe schlägt im Prinzip auch Harari, dessen Position weiter unten noch intensiver zu diskutieren sein wird. Unabhängig von den politischen Folgen – z. B. die fortwährende Diskussion über ein bedingungsloses Grundeinkommen – stellt sich die Frage, ob – im Frankl'schen Sinne – dem Menschen hier im großen Stil Sinnverwirklichungsmöglichkeiten abhanden zu kommen drohen. Oder ob – wie etwa bei Precht – der technologische Fortschritt nicht viel mehr die Möglichkeiten mit sich bringt, den Menschen endlich von vielerlei stupiden und mühsamen Tätigkeiten zu befreien und ihn, ausgestattet mit einem bedingungslosen Grundeinkommen, in einen Zustand der Muße zu versetzen, der es ihm erlaubt, sein Leben schöpferisch so zu gestalten wie er es wirklich will.

Konsens scheint also zu sein, dass die Veränderungen in der Arbeitswelt einschneidend sein werden. Sollten Millionen Menschen ihre Arbeit verlieren und darüber hinaus keinen Zugang zu adäquaten Ersatzbeschäftigungen erhalten, könnte sich nun jene geistige Not wiederholen, die Viktor Frankl schon im letzten Jahrhundert beschrieben hat (Vgl. Frankl 1946/2017: 166 – 178)

Es gibt also Grund zur Annahme, dass der technologische Fortschritt zwar einerseits zu einer Befreiung des Menschen von unangenehmen, monotonen Tätigkeiten führen wird, andererseits aber auch zu einer millionenfachen Freisetzung von Arbeitskräften, die mit der Herausforderung konfrontiert werden, ihrem Leben im schöpferischen Sinne einen neuen Inhalt zu geben.

Was diese Situation nun nochmals dramatisch verschärfen dürfte, ist die weiterhin steigende Lebenserwartung: Die Lebensspanne, welche Menschen außerhalb des Erwerbslebens zur Verfügung steht, wird seit Jahrzehnten immer länger. Sollte sich der Arbeitsmarkt, wie angedeutet, radikal verändern und Millionen Arbeitskräfte freigesetzt werden, wären diese dann womöglich, aufgrund einer weiterhin ansteigenden Lebenserwartung, auch noch mit der Notwendigkeit konfrontiert, viel mehr Jahre als bisher mit *Sinn* in Form von schöpferischen Tätigkeiten zu füllen.

Eine Art Brücke zwischen der Kategorie der Schöpfungswerte und jener der Erlebniswerte bilden Kunst und Kultur. Für die Kunstreibenden handelt es sich um einen schöpferischen Akt, für die Kunstkonsumenten hingegen um die Verwirklichung von Erlebniswerten. Auf den ersten Blick möchte man nun vermuten, dass es sich hierbei um ein Feld handelt, in welchem der Mensch, unberührt von etwaigen technologischen Entwicklungen, unvertretbar bleibt. Doch auch diese Überzeugung darf angezweifelt werden, wenn man bedenkt, dass Algorithmen und Computer heute bereits in der Lage sind, Kunstgegenstände (beispielsweise Gemälde oder klassische Musik) herzustellen, die selbst in den Augen von Kennern kaum von Artefakten menschlicher Urheber zu unterscheiden sind (vgl. Harari 2019: 497–500).

Erlebniswerte: Wenn Frankl unter dieser Wertkategorie sowohl das (Er)leben von Liebe als auch das Sammeln von selbsttranszendenten Erfahrungen fasst, dann kann auch hier im Angesicht der Digitalisierung gefragt werden, wie sich unsere Art zu lieben und miteinander zu leben in Veränderung begriffen ist. Werden wir beispielsweise in Zukunft menschenähnliche Roboter lieben wie wir bisher nur Menschen lieben konnten? Mag es aktuell auch noch reine Science-Fiction sein, so gibt es keinen Grund anzunehmen, dass die Entwicklung neuer Roboter nicht in diese Richtung immer humanoiderer Modelle gehen könnte – alle vorstellbaren Implikationen inbegriffen. Aber auch was das Sammeln selbsttranszendenter Erfahrungen anbelangt, könnten uns in den nächsten Jahrzehnten große Veränderungen bevorstehen. Techniken des „Virtual Life" könnten es beispielsweise möglich machen, zu „verreisen" ohne dabei den Ort zu verlassen, an dem man sich befindet. Mit entsprechender Technologie ausgestattet begeben wir uns auf fiktive Reisen und kommen sonnengebräunt und erholt wieder – allerdings ohne mit anderen Menschen in einem realen Austausch gewesen zu sein oder auch nur unsere Wohnung verlassen zu haben. Und wie schon weiter oben beschrieben, könnte uns zukünftiger Kunstgenuss nicht mehr in die „Seele des Künstlers" schauen lassen, sondern höchstens in die Tiefe von Computeralgorithmen.

Alle diese Andeutungen sollen Argumente dafür aufzeigen, warum die Art und Weise, wie wir bislang über Sinnverwirklichung im Sinne der von Frankl dargestellten Wertkategorien nachgedacht haben, im 21. Jahrhundert einer rasanten Wandlung unterworfen werden könnte. Die daraus entstehenden Implikationen sind mancherorts schon sichtbar. Gleichwohl lässt sich die Frage stellen, ob der Mensch deshalb seiner *Sinnmöglichkeiten* durch die Technik beraubt wird –

oder ob sich lediglich die *Tätigkeiten* verändern, die uns Sinnerfüllung versprechen.

Die Menschheit auf dem Weg zum *Homo Deus*?

In seinem Buch *Homo Deus* stellt Yuval Harari die Behauptung auf, dass der Mensch im 21. Jahrhundert danach strebt, sich zu einem göttlichen Wesen weiterzuentwickeln. Seine Argumentation: Nachdem die Menschheit in den zurückliegenden Jahrhunderten atemberaubende Fortschritte gemacht hat bei der Bekämpfung der „drei großen Menschheitsplagen" Krieg, Hunger und Krankheit (Harari 2019: 9), wird sich unser Blick künftig sukzessive weg von einer rein problemorientierten Beschäftigung mit Fragen des Überlebens und immer weiter hin zu Fragen der Selbstoptimierung und –weiterentwicklung bewegen. Die zentralen Themen lauten: *Glück*, *Unsterblichkeit* und eben *Göttlichkeit*. Die für unseren Zusammenhang spannende Frage lautet nun, was die von Harari sehr eindrücklich beschriebenen möglichen Entwicklungen für Folgen für das auf Frankl beruhende motivationstheoretische Konzept des *Willens zum Sinn* haben könnten – und wie man mit Frankls Theorie Harari antworten könnte.

Unsterblichkeit: Den Fortschritten der modernen Medizin liegt nach Harari die Überzeugung zugrunde, dass der Tod zunächst einmal nicht, wie in der Vergangenheit geschehen, eine Art religiös begründete Voraussetzung für ein jenseitiges Weiterleben ist. Ebenfalls ist er in den Augen der Forscherinnen und Forscher nicht einfach eine Art Bedingung dafür, dass das Leben selbst Sinn erhält (der im Falle von Unsterblichkeit verloren ginge). Der Tod wird hier schlicht als technisches Problem betrachtet, für das es folglich auch eine technische Lösung geben könnte. Ob eine solche Einstellung klug oder vernünftig ist, mag dahingestellt bleiben. Fakt ist aber wohl, dass es genug Interesse des Menschen zu geben scheint, wesentlich länger und gesünder als bisher leben zu können (vgl. ebd.: 39–51).

Glück: Pharmazeutische Produkte, die beim Menschen künstlich Gefühle des Glücks hervorrufen oder zumindest stimmungsaufhellend wirken, sind nun wahrlich keine Neuheit, jedoch geht Harari auch davon aus, dass die Entwicklungen hier im 21. Jahrhundert weitergehen. Antriebsfeder dafür ist für ihn eine offenbare Gleichsetzung von *Glück* mit dem Gefühlszustand des „glücklich seins" (vgl. ebd.: 52–72), was dann wiederum auf ein biochemisches Problem reduzierbar wäre.

Göttlichkeit: Das dritte große Projekt, so Harari, wird letztlich der Versuch der Menschheit sein, sich selbst in den Stand der Göttlichkeit zu erheben, wobei dieses Ziel u. a. die beiden anderen großen Projekte, Glück und Unsterblichkeit, mit enthält. Darüber hinaus geht es um Möglichkeiten, die eigene biologische Grundlage mithilfe von Biotechnologie, Cyborg-Technologie sowie die Produktion von nicht-organischen Lebewesen zu optimieren: „Die Fähigkeit, unseren Körper und unseren Geist umzugestalten, wünschen wir uns vor allem aus einem Grund, nämlich um Alter, Tod und Elend zu entgehen, aber wer kann schon sagen, was wir sonst noch mit dieser Fähigkeit anfangen könnten, wenn wir sie erst einmal haben." (ebd.: 78)

Neben diesen drei hier kurz beschriebenen Großprojekten für das 21. Jahrhundert beschäftigt sich Harari in seinem Buch unter der Kapitelüberschrift „Die Datenreligion" mit einer – aus Frankls Perspektive reduktionistischen – These: Auch organisches Leben, wie das menschliche, folgt in letzter Konsequenz nur biochemischen Algorithmen. „Der Dataismus [...] verweist darauf, dass für die biochemischen wie für die elektronischen Algorithmen genau die gleichen mathematischen Gesetze gelten. Damit reißt der Dataismus die Grenze zwischen Tieren und Maschinen ein und geht davon aus, dass elektronische Algorithmen irgendwann biochemische Algorithmen entschlüsseln und hinter sich lassen werden." (ebd.: 563 f.). Die Folge davon wären nicht nur Computer die menschliches Verhalten, Fühlen, Wollen und Streben restlos entschlüsseln könnten. Es wäre in einem dystopischen Szenario letztlich auch das Ende der Menschheit wie wir diese kennen. Künstliche Intelligenz in Form von Algorithmen würde uns Menschen besser kennen als wir uns selbst. Auch unsere komplexen menschlichen Gehirne mit all der Kreativität, Intuition und Schöpfungskraft, die wir uns gerne als Spezifika zuschreiben, wären durch die nicht-bewusste Intelligenz von datenverarbeitenden Algorithmen ersetz- und übertreffbar. Anhänger der Logotherapie würden hier, wie oben angedeutet, wahrscheinlich nur einen weiteren reduktionistischen Versuch erkennen, also einen Versuch, die Einzigartigkeit des Menschen und seiner geistigen Person auf Phänomene zu reduzieren, die unterhalb der geistigen Dimension liegen, diese aber nicht erklären. Eine subhumane Erklärung humaner Phänomene. Doch so einfach sollte man es sich nicht machen.

Wenn wir an dieser Stelle hypothetisch davon ausgehen, dass Hararis Prognose zutrifft, könnte man nun fragen, wie ein im Kern humanistischer Ansatz wie jener von Viktor Frankl dieses Szenario bewertet. Ja, dieses Szenario von Harari fordert geradezu eine Antwort der Logotherapie heraus, da hier an vielen Stellen deren Menschenbild und Paradigmen infrage gestellt werden. Spannenderweise lassen sich die drei von Harari beschriebenen künftigen Großprojekte der Menschheit nun jeweils einer Wertkategorie bei Viktor Frankl zuordnen: Das

Thema der Unsterblichkeit kann als Herausforderung für die Kategorie der Einstellungswerte gesehen werden, das Thema Glück für die Frankl'schen Erlebniswerte und das Thema Göttlichkeit für die logotherapeutische Kategorie der Schöpfungswerte.

Unsterblichkeit: Frankl spricht von der „tragischen Trias" aus Leid, Schuld und Tod, der niemand entkommen kann (vgl. Frankl 1946/2017: 319 f.). Allen Menschen ist gemein, dass sie früher oder später leiden müssen, schuldig werden und irgendwann sterben müssen. Die Frage, die ihn in diesem Zusammenhang beschäftigt hat: Wie kann man anhand dieser Unvermeidlichkeit Sinn für sein Leben finden? Die Antwort: Indem man – entsprechend der Wertkategorie der Einstellungswerte – sich zu diesen Umständen sinnvoll verhält, indem man eine sinnvolle innere Haltung einnimmt. Was „richtig" oder „sinnvoll" ist, bleibt hier natürlich stark situationsabhängig. Wie würde Frankl nun eine Situation bewerten, in welcher zumindest zwei Aspekte dieser Trias, nämlich *Leid* und *Tod*, durch den technologischen Fortschritt weitestgehend obsolet oder zumindest zeitlich weit nach hinten geschoben werden?

Frankl bediente sich gerne verschiedener Metaphern, um die besondere Bedeutung hervorzuheben, die ihm zufolge dem aufrechten Leiden zukommt. „Leidensfähigkeit" sei, so heißt es, den anderen Fähigkeiten überlegen, da man sich diese Fähigkeit eben erst „erleiden" müsse, während einem die Schöpfungs- und Erlebnisfähigkeiten von Geburt an, beispielsweise als Talente und funktionierende Sinnesorgane mitgegeben wurden (vgl. Frankl 1997a: 31–34). *„Wer auf Leid tritt, tritt höher"*, so hieß es diesbezüglich schon bei Hölderlin. Was also geschieht mit den Menschen, wenn sie aufgrund des vielfältigen technologischen Fortschrittes ihrer Möglichkeiten beraubt werden, sich Leidfähigkeit zu „erleiden"? Eine mögliche Antwort findet man vielleicht in der Analogie zu anderen Zivilisationskrankheiten: Bessere hygienische Bedingungen halfen in den letzten Jahrhunderten dabei, die Ausbreitung von Krankheiten signifikant zu verringern – andererseits ist unser heutiges Immunsystem womöglich auch viel anfälliger als früher, weil wir uns in immer sterileren Umfeldern bewegen, wodurch unsere natürlichen Abwehrkräfte nur unzureichend trainiert werden. Sollten nun die von Harari beschriebenen Szenarien eintreffen, könnten zukünftige Menschen wegen wesentlich geringerer Belastungen als heute in Zustände des Leidens geraten – sei es in physischer wie auch in psychischer Hinsicht. Denn wo die Möglichkeiten zu Leiden abnehmen, nimmt auch die Leidensfähigkeit ab – und wo die Leidensfähigkeit abnimmt, nimmt die Fähigkeit ab, dem Leben mit Hilfe der von Frankl so benannten „Trotzmacht des Geistes" entgegenzutreten.

Eine andere Antwort könnte darin liegen, dieses Szenario gar nicht erst als problematisch für die Theorie Frankls anzusehen: Auch wenn sich die Zukunftsszenarien wie beschrieben einstellen sollten, ist damit nicht gesagt, dass sich etwas an dem grundsätzlichen Umstand ändern würde, dass menschliches Leben nach wie vor durch Leid konstituiert wird. Möglicherweise verändert sich die Qualität des Leidens, vielleicht sogar noch stärker hin zu psychischen Beschwerden. Auf die wiederum mag es auch technische bzw. biochemische Antworten (z. B. immer bessere Pharmazeutika) geben. Aber das Gefühl der Sinnlosigkeit wird damit nicht grundsätzlich aufgehoben. Und schon gar nicht in Szenarien, die auf eine mögliche künftige Unsterblichkeit des Menschen hinauslaufen. Selbst wenn man auch „nur" eine Verlängerung der durchschnittlichen Lebensdauer auf 200 oder 500 Jahre annimmt, würde sich die Frage stellen, was man mit so viel Zeit anfängt und wie man diese – bei schmaler werdenden Möglichkeiten, seine Leidensfähigkeit zu trainieren – dann auch noch sinnvoll füllt.

Und es stellt sich noch eine weitere Frage, die hier ihrerseits potentiell ins Mark der logotherapeutischen Lehre zielt: *Sinnlosigkeit* ist ja ein Zustand, der an ein Gefühl gekoppelt ist. Sinnlosigkeit muss von einem Subjekt empfunden werden. „Das Leiden am sinnlosen Leben" heißt demgemäß auch eines von Frankls bekanntesten Werken (Frankl 1978). Was passiert aber nun, wenn wir das Leiden als Gefühl abschaffen – verschwindet damit nicht auch zwangsläufig die Sinnlosigkeit? Aus heutiger Sicht mag das verstörend und gleichsam utopisch klingen. Aber eine Welt, in der menschenähnliche Lebewesen leben, die nicht mehr in unserem heutigen Vorstellungssinne an Gefühlen der Sinnlosigkeit leiden (bzw. leiden können) lässt sich logisch widerspruchsfrei denken. Gibt es also *Sinnlosigkeit* als Zustand noch, wenn damit kein subjektives Gefühl einhergeht, wenn keiner es mehr empfindet?

Glück: Werfen wir bezüglich des menschlichen Strebens nach Glück nun einen Blick auf die von Frankl beschriebene Kategorie der *Erlebniswerte*. Glück als „glücklich sein" beschreibt ebenfalls einen Gefühlszustand, der von Menschen empfunden wird. Für Viktor Frankl strebt der Mensch aber in erster Linie nicht einfach danach glücklich zu sein, sondern vielmehr danach, einen Grund zu haben, glücklich zu sein. „Glück muss er-folgen und kann nicht er-zielt werden [...]" (Frankl 1997a, 20). Für Riemeyer meinen die Erlebniswerte „[...] das Erlebnis des Schönen, der Wahrheit und der Liebe" (Riemeyer 2002: 180). Es gehe dabei darum, „[...] etwas Wertvolles aus der Welt in sich aufzunehmen und sich damit selbst zu bereichern." (ebd.). Dies kann durch den Genuss von Kunst und Betrachtung der Natur ebenso geschehen wie durch religiöses Erleben und vor allem durch das Erleben von Liebe in einer wahrhaften Begegnung zwischen einem *Ich* und einem *Du* (Frankl zit. n. Riemeyer 2002: 183). Frankl meint, dass gerade die Verwirklichung von Erlebniswerten in der Lage ist, rückwirkend ein ganzes Leben mit Sinn zu erfüllen. „Denn wenn es sich auch nur um einen Augenblick handelt – schon an der Größe eines Augenblicks läßt sich die Größe eines Lebens messen: die Höhe einer Bergkette wird ja auch nicht nach der Höhe irgendeiner Talsohle angegeben, sondern ausschließlich nach der Höhe des höchsten Berggipfels." (Frankl 1946/2017: 92, Hervorhebungen im Original). *Glück*, so kann man zusammenfassend festhalten, stellt für Frankl also im Zusammenhang mit den Erlebniswerten eine Folge wahrhaften Erlebens dar, welches sich einerseits aus persönlichen Begegnungen und Liebe ergibt, andererseits aber auch durch das Aufnehmen des Wahren und des Schönen, wie es uns u. a. in Natur, Kunst und Kultur begegnet.

Man würde Harari nun Unrecht tun, wenn man ihm vorwerfen würde, dass er naiverweise Glück auf einen biochemischen Prozess reduzieren will. Tatsächlich geht es ihm gar nicht darum, einen differenzierten Glücksbegriff zu entwickeln, sondern eine Wahrnehmung auszudrücken, auf welchen Wegen die Menschheit im 21. Jahrhundert versucht, Gefühle des Glücks auf u. a. biochemischem Wege zu erreichen. Er weist aber im gleichen Atemzug darauf hin, dass Glück, neben einer biochemischen Komponente auch eine psychologische Komponente beinhaltet, die sich aus der Erfüllung von Erwartungen ergibt (vgl. Harari 2019: 59 f.). Der Grund warum unsere – im Vergleich zu früheren Zeiten – objektiv besseren Lebensbedingungen (z. B. über Kennzahlen wie gestiegene Lebenserwartung, gesunkene Kindersterblichkeit, bessere Bildung, ausreichend Kleidung und Nahrung usw.) nicht zu einer Explosion an Glücksgefühlen geführt hat, liegt in der Tatsache begründet, dass gleichzeitig immer auch unsere Erwartungen gestiegen sind. Glücksgefühle scheinen sich also nicht unbedingt an objektiven äußeren Maßstäben zu orientieren, sondern vielmehr an der Frage, inwiefern unsere subjektiven Erwartungen und Hoffnungen an das Leben erfüllt werden.

Trotzdem sind seine Anmerkungen zum prognostizierten Fortgang menschlichen Glücksstrebens mit technischen Hilfsmitteln auch für die Lehre der Logotherapie eine Herausforderung. Denn es stellt sich beispielsweise die Frage, ob künftige Menschen, die auf biochemischem Wege ihr Glücksempfinden zu optimieren versuchen, überhaupt noch in der Lage sind, in Anbetracht der oben beschriebenen Möglichkeiten wie Kunstgenuss und Naturbetrachtung in Verzückung zu geraten. Metaphorisch ausgedrückt: Können Menschen, die sich mithilfe von Glückspillen oder elektronischer Gehirnstimulation in einer Art dauerhaftem Glückszustand befinden, sich noch über die Höhen der Gebirgskette freuen, während sie gleichzeitig die Täler des Lebens gar nicht mehr wahrnehmen?

Göttlichkeit: In der Verwirklichung schöpferischer Werte, im Schaffen von etwas, findet der Mensch nach Frankl Sinn und Befriedigung. Wie weiter oben schon beschrieben, sieht sich auch diese Wertkategorie durch verschiedene, von Harari beschriebene Aspekte herausgefordert – insbesondere durch die durch fortschreitende Digitalisierung, Robotisierung und Algorithmisierung befeuerten Umwälzungen am Arbeitsmarkt. Wenn es nun um die von Harari beschriebene Prognose der Selbst-Vergöttlichung des Menschen geht, befinden wir uns auf einer anderen Stufe der Argumentation. Göttlichkeit sei hier nicht als vage metaphysische Eigenschaft zu verstehen. Auch sollte man dabei weniger an einen allmächtigen (christlichen) Gott denken als vielmehr an die alten griechischen Götter oder die hinduistischen Devas: „Unsere Nachfahren werden weiterhin ihre Eigenheiten, Marotten und Schwächen haben, so wie Zeus und Indra sie hatten. Aber sie werden in ganz anderen Dimensionen lieben, hassen, schaffen und zerstören können." (Harari 2019: 79). Im Folgenden möchte ich mich auf die hier genannten Möglichkeiten des *Schaffens* konzentrieren.

Bei Frankl beziehen sich die schöpferischen Werte auf selbsttranszendent zu verwirklichende Werte. Deren Verwirklichung ist nun abhängig von den Fähigkeiten und Talenten, die wir besitzen. Jeder Mensch ist im Sinne der Logotherapie dazu aufgerufen, im Rahmen seiner Möglichkeiten nach Wertverwirklichung im Außen zu streben – durch Werke, die man eben schafft, oder Tätigkeiten, denen man nachgeht. Da unsere Fähigkeiten einerseits beschränkt sind, andererseits sich aber dem Menschen von heute eine Vielzahl an potentiellen Möglichkeiten bieten, schöpferische Werte zu verwirklichen, suchen wir oft nach Orientierung und können am Mangel derselben gegebenenfalls auch verzweifeln. Wenn es nun dazu kommt, dass die Menschheit künftig dazu übergeht, wie weiter oben beschrieben, ihren biologischen Unterbau (z. B. über Genmanipulation) zu optimieren, andererseits aber viele objektive Möglichkeiten der schöpferischen Wertverwirklichung wegfallen, weil Maschinen und Computer diese Aufgaben besser, schneller und günstiger erledigen können, dann könnte das die Brisanz aus logotherapeutischer Sicht nochmal deutlich verschärfen.

Darüber hinaus stellt sich natürlich die Frage, ob Menschen, die sich durch Biotechnologie und Cyborgtechnologie (vgl. Harari 2019: 74) nach göttlichen Fähigkeiten ausstrecken und sich beispielsweise im Laufe eines Lebens immer wieder neu kreieren, überhaupt noch Menschen sind oder ob wir es hier dann bereits mit einer posthumanen Spezies zu tun hätten. Wenn dem so sein sollte, gerät eine humanistisch orientierte Form der Psychotherapie wie die Logotherapie an ihre natürlichen Grenzen.

Quo Vadis, sapiens?

Am Ende von *Homo Deus* stellt Harari drei Fragen, von denen er hofft, dass sich die Leserinnen und Leser weiter damit beschäftigen (vgl. Harari 2019: 608):

1. Sind Organismen wirklich nur Algorithmen, und ist Leben wirklich nur Datenverarbeitung?
2. Was ist wertvoller – Intelligenz oder Bewusstsein?
3. Was wird aus unserer Gesellschaft, unserer Politik und unserem Alltagsleben, wenn nicht-bewusste aber hochintelligente Algorithmen uns besser kennen als wir uns selbst?

Im Frankl'schen Sinne wäre die Bejahung der ersten Frage, wie schon weiter oben erläutert, nichts als eine weitere Variante des Reduktionismus. Andererseits sollte sich die Logotherapie, will sie eine Zukunft haben, mit dieser neuen reduktionistischen Herausforderung intensiv auseinandersetzen. Algorithmen bestimmen schon heute weite Teile des Alltags der Menschen – und schon heute lassen wir uns viele Entscheidungen von ihnen abnehmen. Beispiele dafür wären der Kauf des nächsten Buches bei Amazon, die Wahl eines Partners bei Tinder oder die Entscheidung über die Annahme eines bestimmten Ausbildungsplatzes aufgrund von Persönlichkeits- und Berufswahltests. Noch mag es sich dabei um Randerscheinungen handeln, aber je besser die hier zugrundeliegenden Algorithmen in Zukunft noch werden (und die dafür notwendigen Daten fließen jeden Tag, rund um die Uhr, weltweit), desto wahrscheinlicher wird es, dass wir ihnen auch immer mehr vertrauen. Und im Umkehrschluss vertrauen wir dann unserer eigenen Intuition und unseren Gefühlen (sprich: unseren, von der Evolution hervorgebrachten, Algorithmen) immer weniger. Denn wir machen die Erfahrung, dass uns diese auch schon hier und da mal trügen. Künstliche Algorithmen können nun zwar auch zu falschen oder suboptimalen Ergebnissen in Bezug auf die oben genannten Beispiele führen. Aber im Gegensatz zu unserer natürlichen Intuition, werden künstliche Algorithmen mit rasender Geschwindigkeit besser und treffsicherer.

Kann man aber noch von einem *freien Willen* bzw. von *Freiheit* und *Verantwortung* sprechen, wenn wir diese Verantwortung sukzessive immer öfter gar nicht wirklich selber treffen, sondern letztlich (quasi externen) Algorithmen überlassen, während wir selber nur noch eine bestimmte Taste auf dem Handy drücken und uns damit dem (womöglich trügerischen) Gefühl hingeben, dass wir wenigstens noch diese letzte manuelle Handlung zur Umsetzung einer Entscheidung selbst vollzogen haben?

Auf die zweite Frage könnte man aus logotherapeutischer Sicht antworten, dass Bewusstsein in jedem Falle wertvoller sei als Intelligenz. Frankl lehrte, dass es niemals darauf ankommt, was einer kann, sondern immer nur darauf was einer tut. Oder, angelehnt an eine andere, oft bemühte Metapher: Es kommt nicht auf die Bausteine an, sondern auf den Baumeister (vgl. Frankl 1997a: 109). Tatsächlich scheint die Forschung noch relativ weit davon entfernt zu sein, künstliches Bewusstsein herstellen zu können. Bewusstsein ist aber seinerseits wiederum notwendig, um Sinn und Sinnlosigkeit zu empfinden. Wenn wir Frankl ernst nehmen, dann ist aber genau das die besondere Würde, die menschlichem Leben zukommt. Auf dem Weg zum Sinn ist Intelligenz (sei es die eigene, oder die zur Verfügung stehende künstliche) folglich immer nur ein Mittel zum Zweck – so wie auch Geld, Macht oder Gesundheit.

Die dritte Frage knüpft unmittelbar an die erste Frage an und stellt in gewissem Sinne deren Erweiterung auf die gesellschaftliche Dimension dar. Der Kern ist auch hier die Aussicht auf eine Situation, in der nicht mehr wir Menschen es sind, die aktiv gestaltend unser Leben führen, sondern in welcher wir im Zuge des Dataismus auf präziseres Wissen zurückgreifen können als je zuvor – und gleichzeitig (das ist der eigentliche Punkt) die *bestmögliche Lösung* in jeder Lebenssituation als Antwort mitserviert bekommen. Diese Situation würde natürlich nicht von heute auf morgen eintreten, sondern sich vielmehr schleichend in mal mehr, mal weniger großen Sprüngen ereignen. Algorithmen würden dann auch Entscheidungen treffen, die der Mensch letztlich nur noch bestätigt, weil wir eben eingesehen haben, dass wir hier unterlegen sind. In Analogie zum Schachspiel würde auch für Bereiche wie die Politik oder die Wirtschaft dann gelten, dass man sich zwar lange mit seinem menschlichen Verstand und seiner Intuition überlegen fühlen konnte, sich dieses Zeitalter aber nun dem Ende zuneigt. Es hat zwar einige Jahrzehnte gebraucht, bevor der beste Schachcomputer in der Lage war, den besten menschlichen Schachspieler zu besiegen – aber danach ging es rasend schnell. Heute wäre es töricht, als Mensch einen dieser Superrechner schlagen zu wollen. Wer gegen einen Schachcomputer gewinnen will, sollte sich einen besseren Schachcomputer suchen, der diese Aufgabe übernimmt. Werden wir Menschen uns also in Zukunft nur noch darin unserer Freiheit und unseres freien Willens vergewissern können, indem wir uns bewusst gegen die von Algorithmen vorgeschlagenen Lösungen entscheiden, um der Situation auf diese Art und Weise zu *trotzen?*

Letztlich scheint Harari mit der dritten Frage auf ganz andere, scheinbar viel simplere Fragen abzuzielen: *Was wollen wir? Wie wollen wir eigentlich leben? Wohin soll die Reise gehen?* Originär philosophische Fragen also. Zumindest den Philosophen dürfte daher auch künftig wohl nicht ihr Tätigkeitsfeld abhandenkommen. Ob und welche Rolle die Logotherapie als sinnzentrierte Psychotherapie hier spielen wird, bleibt offen. Anfang der 1970er Jahre meinte Frankl dazu passend: „Jede Zeit hat ihre Neurosen, und jede Zeit braucht ihre Psychotherapie.“ (Frankl 1971: 35). Die Zukunft wird zeigen, welche Psychotherapie der Mensch im Zeitalter des *Homo Deus* benötigen wird – oder auch nicht.

Literatur

Biller K, de Lourdes Stiegeler M (2017) Wörterbuch der Logotherapie und Existenzanalyse von Viktor E. Frankl. Sachbegriffe, Metaphern, Fremdwörter. Budapest: Süddeutsches Institut für Logotherapie und Existenzanalyse.

Brynjolfsson E, McAfee A (2019) The Second Machine Age. Wie die nächste digitale Revolution unser aller Leben verändern wird. Kulmbach: Plassen.

Fortmann H, Kolocek B (Hg.) (2019) Arbeitswelt der Zukunft. Trends – Arbeitsraum – Menschen – Kompetenzen. Wiesbaden: Springer Gabler.

Frankl VE (1946/2017) Ärztliche Seelsorge. Grundlagen der Logotherapie und Existenzanalyse. München: dtv.

Frankl VE (1955) Pathologie des Zeitgeistes. Rundfunkvorträge über Seelenheilkunde Wien: Deuticke.

Frankl VE (1971) Psychotherapie für den Laien. Rundfunkvorträge über Seelenheilkunde, Freiburg im Breisgau: Herder.

Frankl VE (1972) Der Mensch auf der Suche nach Sinn. Stuttgart: Klett.

Frankl VE (1975) Der leidende Mensch. Anthropologische Grundlagen der Psychotherapie. Bern: Huber.

Frankl VE (1978) Das Leiden am sinnlosen Leben. Psychotherapie für heute, Freiburg im Breisgau: Herder.

Frankl VE (1981/1997b) Die Sinnfrage in der Psychotherapie. 7. Aufl., München: Piper.

Frankl VE (1997a) Der Wille zum Sinn. Ausgewählte Vorträge über Logotherapie. 4. Aufl., Bern: Huber.

Frankl VE (1985/1998) Logotherapie und Existenzanalyse. Texte aus sechs Jahrzehnten. Weinheim: Psychologie Verlags Union.

Harari YN (2019) Homo Deus. Eine Geschichte von Morgen. München: C.H. Beck.

Lyotard JF (1979) La conditione postmoderne. Paris: Éditions Minuit.

Precht RD (2018) Jäger, Hirten, Kritiker. Eine Utopie für die digitale Gesellschaft. München: Goldmann.

Riemeyer J (2002) Die Logotherapie Viktor Frankls. Eine Einführung in die sinnorientierte Psychotherapie. Gütersloh: Quell.

Murray Stein

The meanings of “meaning”

Die Bedeutungen von “Bedeutung”

Zusammenfassung: In diesem Artikel diskutiere und kontrastiere ich eine subjektive und eine objektive Auffassung von Bedeutung. Erstere wird als Gefühl registriert („Sinngefühl“); die andere wird als „Offenbarung‘ empfangen oder ist das Ergebnis einer kognitiven Schlussfolgerung am Ende einer Reflexion über den gesamten Kontext eines Ereignisses oder einer Gruppe verwandter Ereignisse. Die Diskussion basiert auf der Jung’schen Psychologie, ihrer Theorie und Praxis. Jungs Schriften über Synchronizität und das Archetypische werden angeführt, um die Bedeutung als transzendent zum Subjekt zu betrachten. Das Argument ist, dass gemeinsame psychologische Bedeutungsverständnisse partiell sind und durch einen Begriff der Transzendenz ergänzt werden müssen.

Schlüsselwörter: Archetyp, C.G. Jung, Sinn, Synchronizität, Transzendenz, Übersinn,

Abstract: In this article I discuss and contrast a subjective and an objective notion of meaning. The first is registered as a feeling (“a sense of meaning”); the other is received as a “revelation” or is the result of a cognitive conclusion to a reflection on the whole context of an event or a cluster of related events. The discussion is grounded in Jungian psychology, its theory and practice. Jung’s writings on synchronicity and the archetypal are adduced to consider meaning as transcendent to the subject. The argument is that common psychological understandings of meaning are partial and need to be supplemented by a notion of transcendence.

Key words: archetype, C.G. Jung, meaning, supreme meaning, synchronicity, transcendence

Introduction

I still remember well first reading Victor Frankl’s inspiring book, “Man’s Search for Meaning”, many years ago when I was a high school student. It left an indelible impression in my memory. Frankl’s story of survival in the death camps and his subsequent creation of logotherapy constitute one of the 20th century’s great stories of human endurance and resilience. His is a theory tested in the fires of

https://doi.org/10.1515/9783110787153-007

extreme experience. As he discovered, a sense of meaning matters – for our very survival. My later interest in psychoanalysis, specifically in Jungian thought and practice, had its earliest inspiration in Viktor Frankl's Man's Search for Meaning and in Freud's Interpretation of Dreams, which I also read in my adolescence. It was with great pleasure, therefore, that I accepted the invitation to speak at this conference on the topic of "Motivation and Meaning." I will do so from the perspective of Jungian psychology, its theory and practice, since this has been my professional location for the past 45 years. To be honest, Jung has been a core part of my personal sense of meaning and has powerfully motivated me to dedicate my professional activities to writing, teaching, and clinical practice in the field of analytical psychology.

To begin, let me pause for a moment and recognize that "meaning" is a word. Following the guidance of Wittgenstein, I will take a look at how this word is used within the context of analytical psychology. In Jungian circles we use the word "meaning" quite a lot. The question is: how do we use it, and what do we intend to say when we use it? Often it is brought into play when we speak of dreams or numinous experiences, but it also comes up in the everyday sense when we speak about relationships, love, work, career, hobbies, and so forth.

In psychological discourse, we usually use the word, "meaning," to refer to a conscious feeling or a subjective judgment. We speak of "a sense of meaning." A certain activity or a general set of ideas and actions gives us "a sense of meaning." To say that "meaning" is a word that refers to a specific feeling is not to diminish its value or importance. Our feelings are what we live with most of the time, and they often govern our choices and decisions about how to live, who to live with, and in general they set the tone of our everyday lives. Psychotherapists spend a lot of time reflecting on feeling with their patients. Feelings make a difference. A "sense of meaning" is a positive feeling and something most people want in their lives.

Sometimes, however, we also speak of "meaning" as archetypal, that is, as transcendent to consciousness, inhering in the collective unconscious and ultimately delivered to the conscious subject by the objective Self. In this sense, meaning is spoken of not as a conscious feeling but an attribute of a psychological constellation whose source lies outside of consciousness.

On the one hand, then, we speak of "meaning" as subjective, as when we say we have "a sense of meaning"; on the other hand, we speak of "meaning" as objective, i. e., as transcendent to conscious feeling or judgment, as when we say that a synchronistic event (a meaningful coincidence) has occurred. One is an immediate feeling in consciousness, and the other is delayed and arrives in consciousness by way of reflection. The second carries a reference to transcendence. Its source transcends the ego and arrives as a gift of grace.

I will reflect on the relation between these two types of meaning. A question to be considered is this: must a subjective "sense of meaning" participate in objective "transcendent meaning" in order to maintain its power of conviction and motivation? Will a subjective sense of meaning be able to sustain itself as motivational without support from a source beyond the limitations of the subject and transcendent to the ego?

I have to say, however, that even the mere suggestion of transcendent meaning is highly problematic for contemporary women and men. By "contemporary" I mean postmodern in sensibility and outlook. We live in an age that has totally banished myth and metaphysics from serious consideration. In postmodernity we can freely play with myth and speculative imagination, but we do not bind our will and destiny to them as people did in other times and places. We look on such affirmations as pre-modern or pathological. We must ask, therefore: can a person find a sustainable sense of meaning, which may require a transcendent anchor, while at the same time actively participating in a culture such as ours that rejects religious symbols and beliefs as points of orientation? On a collective level, we have no master narratives that connect us to the gods, to the infinite, to the eternal. In this cultural situation, what can sustain a sense of meaning for the individual? Will it not collapse – like a transient mood? For many people this is the case.

Analytical Psychology and the problem of meaning

I will speak now of how analytical psychology addresses this problem, and I will use Jung's recorded experiences as a model. I do this because it is in the public record, and so does not violate rules of confidentiality that ordinarily apply to clinical cases.

It is well known that Jung set out on a search for meaning by going on a quest for a myth to live by when, after writing his defining departure from Freud, *Wandlungen und Symbole der Libido*, he confronted himself and starkly realized that he no longer subscribed to the Christian creed or myth. He suddenly found himself in a vacuum of meaninglessness. What followed was the Red Book period, a deep dive into the life of the imagination. It was a sometimes desperate search for what he called "a personal myth" that could provide and sustain a sense of meaning for himself.

What is a personal myth? In general, myth is a collectively accepted narrative structure of image and thought that implies transcendent reference to objective meaning which lies beyond the groping attempts of mere subjectivity. The eternal gods offer finite mortals a point of reference to transcendent meaning that is absolute and not subject to time and change. Myths are like the stars that guide the mariner across the high seas.

A personal myth is an individually experienced structure of image and narrative that also implies transcendence and objective meaning in the background of a subjective sense of meaning. Myth anchors the relative and time-bound subject's sense of meaning in the absolute. A personal myth, like a collective myth, provides a foundational level of certainty and security for a subjective sense of meaning, like the gold bars kept in the vaults of the Swiss federal bank to back up the country's paper currency. Still, the idea of personal myth sounds strange because we generally think of myth as belonging to a group and having a long history to which the individual is an heir.

Toward the beginning of his *Red Book* and at the outset of his journey through the archetypal inner world of imagination, Jung inscribes a key passage that speaks of the topic of meaning. He writes about a conversation with a figure named simply "Soul", a feminine presence who has confronted and questioned him, and has made some demands.

> On the following night I had to write down all the dreams that I could recollect, true to their wording. The meaning of this act was dark to me. Why all this? Forgive the fuss that rises in me. Yet you want me to do this. What strange things are happening to me? I know too much not to see on what swaying bridges I go. Where are you leading me? Forgive my excessive apprehension, brimful of knowledge. My foot hesitates to follow you. Into what mist and darkness does your path lead? Must I also learn to do without meaning? If this is what you demand, then so be it. This hour belongs to you. What is there, where there is no meaning? Only nonsense, or madness, it seems to me. Is there also a supreme meaning? Is that your meaning, my soul?
> (Jung 2009: 137–138)

and

> Was ist, wo kein Sinn ist? Nur Unsinn oder Wahnsinn, so scheint mir. Gibt es auch einen Übersinn? Ist das dein Sinn, meine Seele? (Jung 2017: 148)

This passage sets the stage for all that is to come in The Red Book. Soul demands that he put aside his acquired conscious "sense of meaning" for a time, which would derive from his previous work as a psychiatrist and author and from his family life and friendships. He is being asked to venture into the unknown without the security offered by his professional positions and achievements. There he might discover Soul's meaning, i.e., supreme meaning (*Übersinn*).

I want to call special attention to three key words in this passage: "meaning" (*Sinn*), "nonsense" (*Unsinn*) and "supreme meaning" (*Übersinn*). The first two belong to the conscious world of the narrator (the ego or "I" in the story), who is a middle-aged Swiss psychiatrist and scientific researcher, and the third is suggested by the Soul (a symbolic figure of the collective unconscious, which is portrayed in the text as a woman, and which Jung would name "anima" in his later psychological theory). The narrator in this story ("I") is willing to let go of his limited sense of meaning, even though it throws him into a confused state of mind where nonsense and madness threaten to consume him. But he tentatively trusts that Soul will provide another, or a different, sense of meaning, namely "supreme meaning" (*Übersinn*). This will be an attribute of the personal myth he is seeking to discover in this journey to the interior of the psyche.

Several kinds of meaning

What kind of meaning (*Sinn*) is typically available to the subject? This would be the sort that we find in our everyday lives, as we invest in our activities and relationships. We don't have to search far for it. It is at hand. It comes along with our activities and achievements. If we have a satisfying job, for instance, and do well in it, a sense of meaning will be a side effect. Or if we see our children grow and do well, we will say that participating in family life and contributing to the wellbeing of loved ones gives us a sense of meaning. This type of meaning is a feeling that is derived from our activities.

This sense of meaning has many levels and can imply deep levels in the psyche. A person might say to her therapist: "I went to the exhibition of contemporary art in Basel. I found it very meaningful." She is saying that it caught her interest, that it spoke to her in some way that was of personal significance, perhaps that it reminded her of vaguely felt but profound associations and feelings. It is hard for her to define more clearly what she means by "meaningful," but clearly this has to do with a feeling of the significance of the experience for her. This could be a transitory feeling that will fade in a short while, or it might be something more significant, a deeper sense of meaning. It could even touch on the archetypal level of her psyche. A psychology of deep meaning is a symbolic psychology, a psychology of soul and the depths of the collective unconscious. It speaks of symbols and their powerful, even numinous, effect on our emotions and consciousness. Such feeling experiences can change our lives and send us in new directions. This level of meaning has irrationally-derived motivational power. The meaning here gives us a will to live.

Sometimes, however, the sudden eruption of a sense of meaning in such numinous experience looks, in retrospect, like a psychotic episode. This is especially true when it is not linked to other more mundane aspects of the sense of meaning in life and work. I recall a patient who came to me one day for a therapy session and claimed that he had seen just that morning a number of highly meaningful symbols in the trees around his house. I asked him what he had seen and what this meant to him. He said that he had seen crosses carved into the bark of the trees and that these were signaling his identity as Jesus Christ. Normally he was a polite and somewhat detached church-goer who regularly attended a Protestant church on Sunday mornings: nothing more mystical than that. At this point in his life, he was a retired businessman with a few minor hobbies that he enjoyed to pass the time. But on this day, he smiled at me in a knowing way, believing that I could now too recognize him as Christ. We spoke about this quietly throughout the session, and I neither contradicted nor agreed with him. He did not seem in any danger. When I saw him again a week later, he had returned back to his normal state of consciousness and did not refer to this episode again. It had faded away, and he now once again functioned as a more or less rational person living in the modern secular world. Nevertheless, it is quite possible, even likely, that his identification with the Christ symbol continued to lie dormant in his unconscious and would continue to offer a sense of transcendent meaning in his life, but in a more subdued way. Even if it was extreme, this experience was not pathological in the sense that it interfered with his normal life. He had momentarily been in the grips of a powerful collective mythic symbol to which supreme meaning (*Übersinn*) is attached.

There is a similar episode recorded in The Red Book, when Jung identifies momentarily with the Crucified Christ figure. In retrospect, some 12 years later, Jung interprets this episode in a seminar given to his students and says of it:

> In this deification mystery you make yourself into the vessel, and are a vessel of creation in which the opposites reconcile. The more these images are realized, the more you will be gripped by them. When the images come to you and are not understood, you are in the society of the gods or, if you will, the lunatic society; you are no longer in human society, for you cannot express yourself. Only when you can say, "This image is so and so," only then do you remain in human society. Anybody could be caught by these things and lost in them – some throw the experience away saying it is all nonsense, and thereby losing their best value, for these are the creative images. Another may identify himself with the images and become a crank or a fool. (Jung 1989: 99)

In short: from such experiences a sense of "supreme meaning" can be forged if they are linked to the rest of a person's life and incorporated into a subjective sense of meaning. The more ordinary sense of meaning can apply to anything – to cleaning out closets, to shopping for a dress, to cooking, to mowing the lawn and working in the garden. It is a feeling of pleasure, and it oils the wheels of the psyche like petroleum in the gears of an automobile engine. This mundane sense of meaning signifies that psychic energy is flowing smoothly into everyday life. We say that libido is in progression. Sometimes this is small and seemingly mundane, and sometimes it is more symbolic and even numinous. Here the soul is actively present (the anima is "the archetype of life itself", according to Jung). When the soul is awake and active in our lives, we feel motivated to get up in the morning and go about our business with a positive, even a joyful, attitude.

Consider the opposite situation. A client says to his therapist: "I just can't bear to go to my job anymore. It has no meaning. It is empty, routine, boring. It grinds me down to dust." His work is tedious, and no longer attracts his libido. It has lost its shine and he has fallen out of love with his tasks and the workplace environment. The sense of meaning is absent. This happens frequently. This is what we call "burnout." It is not really a clinical depression, but rather ennui, "acedia." It can get worse and become more general as "sloth," one of the seven deadly sins. This signals the absence of anima in daily life. "The yeast has gone out of the bread of the land," as Karin Blixen writes so movingly in Out of Africa when her beloved is killed in plane crash. Now the libido disappears and flows backward into the unconscious. This is the mode of regression, and it will almost inevitably produce important and meaningful dreams that eventually suggest a new direction in life and bring a new sense of meaning.

The direction of libido fluctuates, and this gives and takes away the sense of meaning in our daily activities. We are dependent on this flow for our sense of meaning. Often, we are helpless in the face of these fluctuations. They come and go as life happens to us.

The person who finds himself in the condition of burnout is the opposite of someone who feels "called," who has a strong and vibrant sense of vocation, who feels that his tasks, even if mundane and routine on the surface, relate to a sense of purpose. This may relate to raising children or working in the executive suite of a large corporation. A sense of vocation motivates a person to go to work every day with energy and a positive feeling about the day ahead. Such a person is in the "flow," as Csikszentmihalyi says. Being in the "flow" indicates energy, motivation, pleasure, and meaning associated with a specific activity. Mathematicians will find it in doing their calculations, lovers in their affairs, physicians in their surgeries.

This is the type of meaning that is available to the subject when psychic energy is flowing progressively and oriented by symbols. It should be noted, however, that this type of meaning is also not created by the subject. The subject receives the sense of meaning as an effect of the libido's flow into actions that draw it forward. Meaning is offered as an effect of the libido's progressive flow; it is a gift. And it can vanish. Love can suddenly or gradually fade away; interest in one's work and the sense of vocation can evaporate in certain circumstances. In psychotherapy we face these situations on a regular basis. Meaning is suddenly lost after an accident or loss, and every possible action seems to be nonsense. There is no longer any motivation to continue along a given path in life. And when it is lost, it becomes strikingly apparent that a sense of meaning is essential for motivation. The subject cannot go on very well without it. Everything seems mechanical. It is non-sense (*Unsinn*).

In search of a personal myth

This was Jung's condition when he lost his relationship with Freud, as he recounts in *Memories, Dreams, Reflections:* "After the parting of the ways with Freud, a period of inner uncertainty began for me. It would be no exaggeration to call it a state of disorientation. I felt totally suspended in mid-air..." (Jung 1961: 170). It was at this moment that he asked himself:

> In what myth does man live nowadays? In the Christian myth, the answer might be, 'Do you live in it?' I asked myself. To be honest, the answer was no. For me it is not what I live by.' 'Then do we no longer have any myth?' "No, evidently we no longer have any myth.' 'But then what is your myth, the myth in which you do live?' At this point the dialogue with myself became uncomfortable, and I stopped thinking. I had reached a dead end.
> (Jung 1961: 171)

This was the beginning of his search for meaning at midlife.

As we saw in the Red Book experience quoted above, Jung was asked by "Soul" to recall and write down his dreams. At first he did not understand why he should do this. It seemed like nonsense, irrelevant, silly – in other words, meaningless. Nevertheless, he complied with Soul's instruction and did record two important dreams from his childhood. They are recorded in his autobiography, *Memories, Dreams, Reflections:*

> I was in a dark wood that stretched along the Rhine. I came to a little hill, a burial mound, and began to dig. After a while I turned up, to my astonishment, some bones of prehistoric

> animals. This interested me enormously, and at that moment I knew: I must get to know nature, the world in which we live, and the things around us.
>
> There came a second dream. Again I was in a wood; it was threaded with watercourses, and in the darkest place I saw a circular pool, surrounded by dense undergrowth. Half immersed in the water lay the strangest and most wonderful creature: a round animal, shimmering in opalescent hues, and consisting of innumerable little cells, or of organs shaped like tentacles. It was a giant radiolarian, measuring about three feet across. It seemed to me indescribably wonderful that this magnificent creature would be lying there undisturbed, in the hidden place, in the clear, deep water. It aroused in me an intense desire for knowledge, so that I awoke with a beating heart. These two dreams decided me overwhelmingly in favor of science, and removed all my doubts. (Jung 1961: 85 ff.)

These dreams, as he says, instilled his motivation to pursue science over philosophy in his studies and later in his career. Writing them down again, now at the age of 38, reminded him of his vocation as a scientist.

Without doubt, the sense of vocation is one of the most important sources of a sense of meaning in a person's life. It is a great motivator. Vocation is a calling, and the Caller is the Self. The subject receives a calling from a source beyond itself, an inner source that is irrational. In religious language, the Caller is God. This anchors the subject's personal sense of meaning in supreme meaning. People do things out of an emergent sense of vocation that often they cannot explain or justify. They say they simply must do them. Recalling these dreams of his youth brought Jung back to the sense of vocation that had guided him to a meaningful life up to this point. But now he needed something more, something specific and attuned to his present situation. It now became a matter of finding a new path where the old one had given out, but along the same vocational lines. Jung would always be a physician and a scientist, but he had to readjust his vision. He needed to find a myth that could anchor his future work in supreme meaning. His personal sense of meaning from here on forward would depend upon it.

In speaking of searching for "a myth to live by", we are taking a step further on the quest for a sense of meaning. We are looking for a higher-order structure, for what the Red Book refers to as "supreme meaning" (*Übersinn*). What is this "supreme meaning"? It would seem to be something transcendent.

There often comes a moment in life, usually around midlife as it did in Jung's case, when many things that once had a sense of meaning now seem like nonsense, outgrown and lacking in the meaning they once had. This is not exactly the same as burnout, which can often be resolved with some rest and time out. It can instead be an ongoing crisis that needs considerable time and inner work to become resolved. One is not approaching the problem as solvable on the same level. It implies a new starting point on the level of archetype, not of ego. This takes time to emerge from the collective unconscious. In the meantime, there is liminality, a period of waiting and watching what appears in dreams and other irrationally motivated and directed experiences. In this situation, Jung chose to listen to "the spirit of the depths" and not "the spirit of this time." In other words, he looked inward and began his journey through the unconscious by way of active imagination.

This same thing happens to entire collectives or cultures as well as to individuals. Symbol systems, i.e., myths, that at one time in history carried vast collective and transcendent meaning for people lose their numinosity and become nothing more than dead artefacts, cultural curiosities, antiquities, even embarrassments. This is what has happened in the West over the last couple of centuries to the traditional religions. The deep reservoir of meaning offered by the Christianity and its symbols has dried up. The priceless paintings hung on the walls of the great cathedrals are admired for their artistic value, aesthetically, but they no longer induce mystical states of contact with the Divine. The great cathedrals of the Middle Ages have become museums. The sense of supreme meaning once resident in them has vanished, and while the paint remains on the altars and the canvases, the soul has fled elsewhere. This has thrown Western postmodern culture in a state of liminality: "liquid modernity," as Zygmunt Bauman has called it. We are afloat in this milieu as we search for new guiding myths and collective narratives that will offer a sense of supreme meaning.

Myth in our time

This phenomenon of transcendent meaning "fading away" from collective consciousness has happened to religions of the world in many times and places. When the numinosity of ancient pagan religions faded into curious metaphors that held little conviction, Christianity filled the void and offered a new set of symbols that offered a sense of transcendent meaning. Today in Europe and North America, many of the churches and cathedrals of Christendom are museums, collections of aesthetic objects like stained glass windows and beautifully carved altars. They draw tourists but not worshippers. The soul has left and gone elsewhere in search of meaning. What does a culture do when transcendent meaning has left, when it is hollowed out, and nothing is left but concerns about material comfort and entertainment?

For individuals and collectives this spells a time of crisis. We are in such a time in our cultural history Modernity prepared the way and postmodernity has advanced it. Sports events have much more meaning for many people than religious rituals. In a sense, they are religious rituals in secular dress and have some temporary meaning-giving effect, but a sense of transcendent meaning is absent. This means it must be repeated over and over again to maintain its meaning-giving power. Today's football victory becomes a stale memory tomorrow. In the 19th century the numinous left religion for many people and passed over into art. "God is dead," was pronounced, but Richard Wagner's operas carried the aura of the numinous and the theater at Bayreuth became a place of worship. Today the great art museums in New York, London, and Paris act as cathedrals, and so do shopping malls. What they do not claim explicitly, however, and cannot in our postmodern times, is transcendent meaning. In postmodernity, transcendence is a mere idea, and mostly a severely suppressed one.

Übersinn, however, is transcendent meaning. It is objective, not subjective. It is beyond "a sense of meaning." This is meaning that exists beyond the realm of conscious understanding. It may be delivered by symbols. Symbols express meaning that cannot be articulated by the intellect. They are windows to the soul. Do we have such experiences today? Peter Berger wrote of "signals of transcendence," moments of symbolic meaning that happen spontaneously, unannounced and unexpected, anywhere and at any time. This was also Rudolf Otto's experience. In the numinous experience he sensed an invisible power, a *mysterium tremendum et fascinans*.

I recall the dream of a young man who came to me for some sessions of analysis. He had been an orphan and was adopted at the age of 4 by a childless couple. Now at the age of 30 he was struggling with the question of meaning and vocation. He was uncertain about his direction. Then he brought a dream to a session in which he was visiting Istanbul and was in the magnificent Hagia Sophia, a place he had actually experienced on a trip not long before the dream. As he was walking in the cathedral under the dome, he looked up and saw the heavenly scene of the Father God surrounded by other figures. Then he saw the Father coming lower in the dome and he felt himself ascending. As they approached one another, the Father looked him in the eye, pointed his finger toward him, and said in a grave voice that echoed throughout the space: "I want you!" The young man woke with tears in his eyes. As he told me the dream, we both had tears in our eyes. He felt "chosen," as he had been chosen at the age of four by his adoptive parents. Only now the figure choosing him was transcendent, and this would become a ground for his personal myth as he went forward into the rest of his life. A pattern was repeating itself in his life: being chosen.

Jung found a way of theorizing about transcendent meaning in his writings on synchronicity. Jung defined synchronicity as a "meaningful coincidence," a convergence of an inner event like a dream or intuition and an outer event. He gives a number of examples of this from his clinical practice. Inevitably these coincidences struck the chord of a type of meaning that is not manmade or constructed. What type of meaning is this? Not all coincidences are meaningful, but when they are, the element of meaning is delivered by the convergence of causally unrelated events and is perceived by the subject as having meaning. Jung speaks of synchronicity as a special case of "acausal orderedness" (Jung 1969: par. 965), which includes "factors such as the properties of natural numbers and the discontinuities of modern physics." He continues: "...we must regard them as creative acts, as the continuous creation of a pattern that exists from all eternity, repeats itself sporadically, and is not derivable from any known antecedents" (Jung 1969: par. 967). The meaning contained in synchronistic events is in the pattern that is anchored in a transcendent process of creativity, which is repeated in time unpredictably. From Jung's account in his writings, including his autobiography, we can see that he considered synchronicity to be an essential element in the creation of a personal myth, a myth to live by. Behind synchronicity lay the self as "the archetype of orientation and meaning [...]. For me, this insight signified an approach to the center and therefore to the goal. Out of it emerged a first inkling of my personal myth" (Jung 1961: 199). This realization of a personal myth was backed by a number of synchronicities that anchored it securely in "supreme meaning."

In Jungian work, the process of forming a personal myth is made up of a combination of passive waiting ("Wu wei", as the Taoist masters call it) and active engagement with dreams, images and synchronistic events. The subject arrives at the sense of meaning, personal and transcendent, by paying careful attention to these data. It is a process with many ups and downs, twists and turns. "The way is serpentine," as Jung describes the individuation journey. It includes sense and nonsense and supreme meaning, and at any given moment we can be in touch with any one of these meanings of meaning.

Conclusion

I would like to close this talk with a passage from *Memories, Dreams, Reflections* that speaks in moving terms of the meaning of human consciousness itself within the cosmos. In this reflection, Jung gives humankind a standing that is coequal with the Creator. The human contribution has to do with the realization of meaning in nature. This would also speak to our ecologically sensitive time.

In the chapter titled "Travels," Jung tells of his experiences in many parts of the world outside Europe, and among them is his account of his journey in 1925 to Kenya and Uganda. Toward the beginning of that trip, he had the opportunity to step out of the company he was with and take some time apart and alone. He writes:

> I walked away from my companions until I had put them out of sight, and savored the feeling of being entirely alone. There I was now, the first human being to recognize that this was the world, but who did not know that in this moment he had first really created it... There the cosmic meaning of consciousness became overwhelmingly clear to me. "What nature leaves imperfect, the art perfects," say the alchemists. Man, I, in an invisible act of creation put the stamp of perfection on the world by giving it objective existence.... Now I knew... that man is indispensable for the completion of creation that, in fact, he himself is the second creator of the world, which alone has given to the world its objective existence – without which, unheard, unseen, silently eating, giving birth, dying, heads nodding through hundreds of millions of years, it would have gone on in the profoundest night of non-being down to its unknown end. Human consciousness created objective existence and meaning, and man found his indispensable place in the great process of being. (Jung 1961: 255–256)

In this quiet moment, and alone in the vast savannah, Jung discovered the meaning of human consciousness and tied it into his sense of supreme meaning within the cosmic structure of Creation itself. This, too, became an important piece in his myth of meaning. One could argue that it might provide a basis for a collective myth of meaning for all of humanity in our time. Humans are not existent because of meaningless chance, and as such even a blight and a cancer on the face of our planet. We are here to bring the world to consciousness. This is our meaning in the great scheme of things. It is up to us to do something of significance with this sense of supreme meaning.

References

Jung CG (2009) The red book. New York: W.W. Norton.
Jung CG (2017) Das Rote Buch. Patmos Verlag.
Jung CG (1989) Analytical psychology. Princeton: Princeton University Press.
Jung CG (1961) Memories, dreams, reflections. New York: Vintage.
Jung CG (1969) Synchronicity: An acausal connecting principle. In *Collected works of C.G. Jung*, vol. 8. Princeton: Princeton University Press.

Felix Tretter

„Der Wille zum Sinn“ – ökosystemtheoretische Aspekte

The will to meaning – ecosystem theoretical aspects

Zusammenfassung: „Sinn“ ist vor allem im Kontext der Psychotherapie und der Psychiatrie von besonderer praktischer Bedeutung, insofern manche Menschen, insbesondere mit depressiven Syndromen, eine Sinnkrise zeigen. Und umgekehrt: der Verlust von „Bezugsobjekten“, insbesondere im sozialen Bereich, wie etwa durch den Verlust der Arbeit oder gar durch Verlust eines geliebten Menschen, kann bei jedem Menschen zu depressiven Symptomen und Sinnkrisen im Leben führen, mit der Frage „Wozu das alles, was soll ich tun?“ In dem Beitrag wird vorgeschlagen, einen grundlegenden „ökosystemischen“ Blick auf das Sinnphänomen zu werfen, bei dem Umweltbeziehungen der Person und deren systemische Struktur betrachtet werden.

Wenngleich der Sinnbegriff sehr heterogen konstruiert ist, wird unter Bezug auf das Sinnkonzept von Viktor Frankl versucht, wegen der Situationsbezogenheit von Sinnphänomenen und der Situiertheit des Menschen, einen *humanökologischen Rahmen* aufzuzeigen. Für detailliertere strukturtheoretische Betrachtungen erscheinen im Anschluss daran Ansätze der *Systemwissenschaft* nützlich: Sinn wird demnach zunächst auf den *erlebten Konsistenzgrad* der Struktur des Netzwerks der Elemente affektiv-kognitiver Repräsentationen zurückgeführt. Sinnfindung und Sinnverlust werden daran anknüpfend, aber globaler als nichtlineare Dynamik in der synergetischen *Potenziallandschaft* von Systemzuständen interpretiert. Schließlich wird ein für die Praxis nutzbares einfaches *Regelkreismodell* von Sinn als Wertesystem vorgeschlagen, das psychische Störungen, wie Depressionen, besser verstehen lässt.

Weitere interdisziplinäre Fachdiskurse müssten allerdings die Adäquatheit, die Relevanz und die Grenzen dieser „ökosystemischen Perspektive“ überprüfen.

Schlüsselwörter: Situiertes Subjekt, Sinn und Umwelt, Ökopsychologie, strukturelle Konsistenz, Sinn als Attraktor, Regelkreismodell und Sollwert

Abstract: “Meaning” is of particular and practical importance, especially in the context of psychotherapy and psychiatry, insofar as some people, especially with depressive syndromes, exhibit a crisis of meaning. And vice versa: the loss of “objects of reference”, especially in the social sphere, such as the loss of work

https://doi.org/10.1515/9783110787153-008

or even the loss of a loved one, can lead to depressive symptoms and crises of meaning in life in any person, with the question "Why all this, what should I do?" The paper proposes to take a basic "ecosystemic" view of the meaning phenomenon, looking at environmental relationships of the person and their systemic structure.

Although the concept of meaning is constructed in a very heterogeneous way, with reference to Viktor Frankl's concept of meaning, an attempt is made to show a human ecological framework because of the situationality of meaning phenomena and the situatedness of the person. For more detailed structural theoretical considerations, approaches of systems science appear useful afterwards: According to this, meaning is first traced back to the experienced degree of consistency of the structure of the network of elements of affective-cognitive representations. Following on from this, but more globally, sense-making and sense-loss are interpreted as nonlinear dynamics in the synergetic potential landscape of system states. Finally, a simple closed-loop model of meaning as a value system that can be used in practice is proposed to better understand mental disorders, such as depression.

However, further interdisciplinary professional discourse would need to examine the adequacy, relevance, and limitations of this "ecosystemic perspective."

Keywords: Situated subject, meaning and environment, ecopsychology, structural consistency, meaning as attractor, control loop model and set point

Semantische Differenzierung und Integration des Sinnbegriffs

Der Ausdruck „Sinn“ findet sich in verschiedenen sprachlichen Verwendungszusammenhängen, etwa als Bezeichnung für die einfache semantische „Bedeutung“, für „Schlüssigkeit“ und „Ordnungsstiftung“, aber auch als Präferenz bzw. Relevanz in Form von „Wertigkeit“, „Wichtigkeit“ (Lampersberger 2014). Systematisch betrachtet sind auch die Prozess-Aspekte *Sinnsuche, Sinnfindung, Sinngebung, Sinnverlust* zu berücksichtigen. Darüber hinaus betreffen Bezeichnungen wie *Sinnbezirke*, *Sinnsucht*, *Wahnsinn*, aber auch *Unsinn*, usw. wichtige Bedeutungsdimensionen dieses Begriffs, mit Gemeinsamkeiten und Unterschieden. Man erkennt damit zugleich, dass Sinn wohl nur für Menschen „Sinn macht“, denn Computern kann man Sinnsuche über die rein semantische Sinnsuche bei Zeichenketten schwerlich zuschreiben.

Diese Vielfalt der umgangssprachlichen, aber auch fachsprachlichen Deutungen macht es somit schwer, eine Basis für eine präzise interdisziplinäre Verständigung über diesen äußerst grundlegenden Begriff herzustellen.

Für den hier interessierenden klinischen Kontext der Psychiatrie und Psychotherapie ist allerdings die disziplinübergreifende Ausarbeitung des Sinn-Konzepts durch den Neurologen, Psychiater, Psychotherapeuten und Philosophen Viktor Frankl zur Existenzanalyse und Logotherapie richtungsweisend (Frankl 1994; Frankl 1997a; Frankl 1997b; Längle 2005). Im Zentrum seiner Arbeiten wird nämlich zunächst grundlegend die *anthropologische Dimension* des Sinnbegriffs erfasst und daran anknüpfend eine konkrete nachhaltige Arbeitsperspektive für Menschen, die mit Menschen arbeiten, aufgezeigt. Frankl betont dabei, dass der *Mensch als Person erst im Verstehen* und *Verwirklichen von Werten zu sich selbst gelangt*, sodass Werte als Sinngeber theoretisch, empirisch und praktisch zu einem zentralen Element menschlichen Daseins und Erlebens werden. Darüber hinaus betont er den Umweltbezug als wesentliches Bestimmungsmerkmal des Sinnbegriffs, vor allem in existenziellen Extremsituationen (Frankl 1997a: 34):

> Sobald menschliches Dasein nicht mehr über sich selbst hinausweist, wird Am-Leben-Bleiben sinnlos (...)

Auch einer der einflussreichsten Schüler von Frankl, Alfried Längle, betont die ein Einzelerlebnis übergreifenden Bedeutungs-Zusammenhänge, die auch den Umweltbezug, also den Situationsbezug, der Sinnfrage betreffen (Längle 1988: 40):

> Jede Situation geht den Menschen persönlich an, meint ihn, spricht ihn an, ruft ihn an, wobei alles nur darauf ankommt, nur wach genug zu sein, den Anspruch der Situation zu vernehmen. Dieses Wechselspiel zwischen Anspruch der Situation (logos) und Antwort der Person fundiert mit ihrem dialogischen Charakter die menschliche Existenz.

Ähnlich, aber stärker ökologisch und systemisch orientiert, formulieren diesen Person-Situations-Bezug Günter Kinast und Maria Fischer (Kinast u. Fischer 1999: 88 f.):

> ... einen Sinn erkennen heißt, eine Ganzheit zu erfassen bzw. uns in Zusammenhängen zu verstehen. Somit ergibt sich Sinn durch die Selbsteinbindung der Person in ein größeres Ganzes, in ein soziales Gefüge (Mitwelt), in die Natur (Umwelt) oder auch in eine Idee.

Über diese Aspekte hinaus kann – vom Kleinen zum großen Ganzen hin – der Sinn eines Erlebnisses, einer Handlung, eines Lebensabschnitts und des ganzen Lebens unterschieden werden (Lampersberger 2014: 9).

Diese hier hervorgehobenen Charakterisierungen lassen gut erkennen, dass die Sinnthematik eine äußere Umweltbezogenheit für den Menschen impliziert. Sinn betrifft in dieser Hinsicht also die *Mensch-Umwelt-Beziehungen*, die Gegenstand des Forschungsprogramms der *Humanökologie* sind. Wegen der Komplexität dieses Beziehungsgefüges, vor allem im Erleben der betreffenden Person und was den Konsistenzaspekt dieser Strukturen betrifft, ist darüber hinaus, zumindest für die wissenschaftliche Analyse, die *Systemperspektive* nützlich. Beide Sichtweisen, die humanökologische und die systemtheoretische, die grundlegend über die System-Umwelt-Dialektik miteinander verwoben sind, können hier – jedoch nur aspekthaft – angesprochen werden. Allerdings wird an dieser Stelle bereits eine philosophische Grundproblematik deutlich, nämlich die Frage, inwieweit die Umwelt „objektiv“ oder nur „subjektiv“ vorhanden ist, was ja das Gelingen einer psychiatrisch-psychotherapeutischen kommunikativen Praxis wesentlich bestimmt.

Die objektive und die subjektive Situation – epistemologische Aspekte

Ausgehend von dem klinischen Beispiel, dass Menschen mit signifikanten Verlusterfahrungen reaktiv-depressive Syndrome und Suizidtendenzen entwickeln können und dann Sinndefizite in ihrem Leben beklagen, deren „Behandlung“ für Therapeuten schwierig sind, soll hier zunächst die Frage angesprochen werden, wie „wirklich die Wirklichkeit“ ist (Watzlawick 1976). Diese Frage wurde von Konstruktivisten weitgehend so beantwortet, dass die Welt oder eine einzelne Situation eine individuelle und soziale Konstruktion ist, und dass wir nur herausfinden können, ob diese Konstruktionen „viabel“ sind (Maturana & Varela 1987; Glasersfeld 1996). Diese Individuum-zentrierte Sichtweise wird unter anderem durch Befunde aus der (visuellen) Wahrnehmungsforschung, wie der Gestaltpsychologie, gestützt, die zeigen, dass eine Anordnung von Einzelreizen als Gestalt wahrgenommen wird, und zwar ohne Zutun des Bewusstseins. Auch in Schwarz-Weiß-Mustern, die zunächst zufällig arrangiert anmuten, kann nach Hinweisen beispielsweise ein Dalmatiner-Hund wahrgenommen werden, was zeigt, dass es im Wahrnehmungssystem unbewusste Gestaltgeneratoren gibt. Allerdings zeigen derartige experimentelle Ergebnisse auch, dass bestimmte Reizkomponenten vorhanden sein müssen, damit ein ganzes Bild wahrgenommen wird, dass also eine externe Realität eine notwendige, aber offensichtlich nicht hinreichende Bedingung für die Objekt-Wahrnehmung ist. Das bedeutet, dass die individuell-subjektive Umweltwahrnehmung sowohl konstruiert ist wie auch von der objektiv bzw. intersubjektiv verifizierten Realität abhängt.

Diese Doppelseitigkeit der Welterfahrung spiegelt sich auch in der philosophischen Kontroverse der ersten Person-Perspektive versus der Dritten-Person-Perspektive, die als Qualia-Problem bekannt ist (Nagel 1974). Die Differenz in der Frage, ob die „Umwelt“ da draußen oder drinnen im Kopf des Betrachters „ist“, erscheint nicht auflösbar und bedeutet, grundlegend auf die Erkenntnistheorie bzw. Wissenschaftstheorie der Human- und Sozialwissenschaften bezogen, dass eine hybride Position erforderlich ist. Ein „konstruktiver Realismus“ (Wallner 1992) bzw. ein „wissenschaftlicher Realismus“ (Psillos 1999) erscheint daher als Mischform am passendsten.

Vor allem in der hier interessierenden *ökologischen Psychologie* als Bereich der Humanökologie der Person wurde diesbezüglich, und zwar auf den Lewin'schen Begriff „Lebensraum“ zentriert, bereits zwischen Kurt Lewin und Egon Brunswik eine tiefgreifende Debatte geführt (Lewin 1951). Die hybride Situation, dass die subjektive und die objektive Beschreibung der (sozialen) Umwelt unauflösbar ist, wurde auch von dem bedeutenden Soziologen Pierre Bourdieu anerkannt (Bourdieu 2004). Auch in der psychiatrisch-psychotherapeutischen Praxis macht die Differenz zwischen „objektiver“ Expertensicht auf die Welt und „subjektiver“ Sicht von Klient*innen das zentrale Spannungsfeld aus, das vor allem bei depressiven und wahnhaften Syndromen herausfordernd ist (Abb. 1).

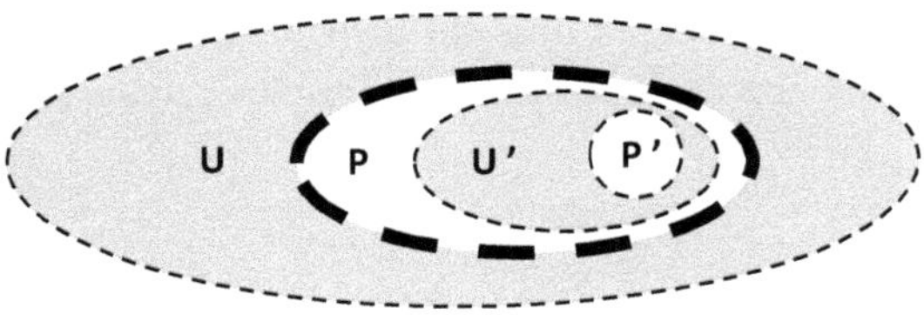

Abb. 1: Die Doppelperspektive der „Ökologie der Person“: die objektive äußere Umwelt U und die subjektive verinnerlichte Umwelt U' als individuelle repräsentative Konstruktion der Umwelt der Person P mit dem Bild der Person von sich selbst (Selbstbild P') und den P-U-Verhältnissen (als relative Größen)

Die humanökologisch-systemische Perspektive zum Sinn-Phänomen

Die Feststellung, dass es schwerlich möglich ist, allein aus sich selbst einen Sinn zu finden, sondern dass die Umwelt, bzw. die Situation als Umweltbezug, dafür sehr wichtig ist, wirft die Frage auf, wie dieser Doppelaspekt wissenschaftlich belastbar aufgefangen werden kann. Dazu wird hier vorgeschlagen, die *ökologische Psychologie* (Lewin et al. 1936; Lewin 1951; Brunswik 1956; Barker 1968; Gibson 1977; Bronfenbrenner 1997) bzw. die *Humanökologie* in Form einer „Ökologie der Person" (Tretter 2008) zu nutzen. Dieses Gebiet soll hier zunächst kurz charakterisiert werden

Humanökologie und ökologische Psychologie

Humanökologie ist der wissenschaftliche Versuch, die verschiedensten Ansätze zur Analyse der *Mensch-Umwelt-Beziehung*, also Umweltübernutzung, Umweltbelastung usw., wie sie aus geophysikalischer, biologischer, psychologischer oder soziologischer Sicht bestehen, zu einer umfassenden Perspektive, gewissermaßen als Plattform der Fachdisziplinen, zusammen zu führen (Knötig 1976; 1979; Glaeser 1989; Glaeser & Teherani-Krönner 1993; Serbser 2004). Diese umweltbezogene Perspektive wurzelt historisch im bioökologischen Ansatz, wie er von Ernst Haeckel ursprünglich explizit formuliert wurde (Haeckel 1866), sie wurde aber in den Humanwissenschaften in der Form der Populationsökologie in der Soziologie der Städte mit der Untersuchung von Raum-Bevölkerungsverhältnissen angewendet (Park et al. 1925).

Im Bereich der Individualwissenschaften wie der Psychologie entwickelte sich, wie erwähnt, die ökologische Psychologie, die im Wesentlichen auf der topologischen Psychologie von Kurt Lewin beruht und auf dem Begriff „Lebensraum" aufbaut und als theoretisches Konstrukt die Person-Umwelt-Beziehungen abbildet (Lewin 1951).

Der Lebensraum und Zielbezug als Sinn

Das Konzept Lebensraum, das die Person-Umwelt-Beziehungen aus psychologischer Sicht erfassen soll, umfasst verschiedene Lebensbereiche als Feldsegmente und vor allem das Leben der Menschen als Zeitpfeil (Vektor): Beispielsweise wird das attraktive Ziel der Person, in Zukunft ein Arzt sein zu wollen, durch das auf dem Weg dahin als Barriere wirkende Medizinstudium abgepuffert. Das Ziel hat eine *positive Valenz*, das Studium eine *negative Valenz*. Das Verhältnis der Valenzen zueinander ergibt eine *Inkonsistenz* und in ihrer Wirkung eine *Ambivalenz* für die Person. So kann es (individuell) „sinnlos" sein, Medizin zu studieren, weil das Studium, aus verschiedenen individuellen Gründen, zu schwer zu realisieren sein mag. Ganz allgemein gesagt, und unter Bezugnahme auf die Philosophie, lässt sich – wenn man in diesem Modell den Zielbereich dieses Vektors grundlegend als Endpunkt kennzeichnen will – das Erreichen dieses Endpunkts als eine Facette eines „gelungenen Lebens" bezeichnen (Abb. 2).

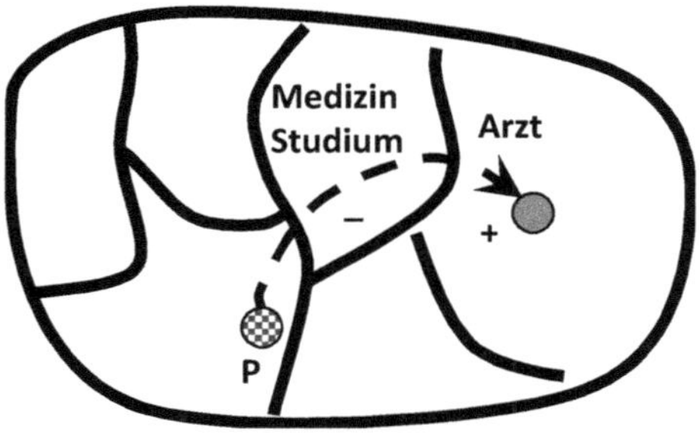

Abb. 2: Die inneren Repräsentationen der individuellen Welt als „Lebensraum" im Modell der topologischen Psychologie mit durch Barrieren getrennten Lebensbereichen und ihren unterschiedlichen Valenzen (-/+) für die Person P.

Im Rahmen des Konzepts vom Lebensraum und auf der Grundlage der Annahme der Situiertheit der Person in eine individuelle, aber auch kollektiv geteilte Lebenslage lässt sich eine Grunddynamik annehmen, die dem Leben die Bewegung in der Zeit und im Raum verleiht. Damit wird bei der Analyse grundlegend vom Leben als eine gerichtete Größe, also einem *Vektor*, ausgegangen, was auch mit Ausführungen von Alfried Längle zur Konstruktion des Sinnbegriffs von Frankl zusammenpasst (Längle 2005).

Anzumerken wäre hier noch, dass dieses Konzept in seiner Konstruktion auch eng mit jenem der „Strukturdynamik" des Psychiaters Werner Janzarik korrespondiert: Auch er geht von einem Feldkonzept des Psychischen aus und sieht „Gerichtetheiten" der psychischen Dynamik, die von der psychischen Struktur geprägt sind und pathologische Entgleisungen bedingen können (Janzarik 1988). Psychosen mit ihren eigenweltlichen Sinnstrukturen sind dann als dynamikbedingte Verwerfungen der Struktur zu verstehen, die ihrerseits wieder die Dynamik verändern. Dieser Doppelaspekt wird hier später im Rahmen der Synergetik nochmals systemtheoretisch angedacht.

Humanökologische Differenzierung des Umweltbegriffs

Die Frage, was denn unter „Umwelt" bzw. „Situation" zu verstehen ist, zeigt bereits eine bemerkenswerte Vielfalt, wie es das eben dargestellte ökopsychologische Modell des Lebensraums verdeutlicht. Es findet teilweise eine Entsprechung in der Soziologie, etwa in Form des Konstrukts „Lebenswelt" von Alfred Schütz (Schütz & Luckmann 1975). Auch hierbei handelt es sich um ein grundlegendes Subjekt-bezogenes Konstrukt der sozialen Umwelt. Bezugnehmend darauf wird von dieser phänomenologischen Schule auch der Sinnbegriff als konstitutiv für die Soziologie dargestellt. Demnach ist das Konstrukt Lebenswelt auch für praktische Handlungsfelder – etwa für Pädagogen und Sozialpädagogen – nützlich (Mühlum et al. 1986; Oppl & Weber-Falkensammer 1986; Thiersch 2015).

Diese Umwelt-bezogenen Begriffe bilden grundlegende Theorie-Bausteine für eine umfassendere Ökologie des Menschen, also einer Individuum-zentrierten Form der „Humanökologie" (Tretter & Löffler-Stastka 2019). In diesem Fachkontext hat sich ein differenzierter Gebrauch des Ausdrucks „Umwelt" entwickelt, der auch für weitere theoretische Differenzierungen des Sinn-Begriffs nützlich zu sein scheint.

Im Gegensatz zur diversifizierten fachsprachlichen Konstruktion des Umweltbegriffs und zu seinem vagen Gebrauch in der Alltagssprache wurde nämlich im Kontext der ökologischen Humanwissenschaften der semantischen Struktur des Umweltbegriffs grundlegend mehr Aufmerksamkeit gewidmet. Zunächst ist – wie vorher ausgeführt – nicht pauschal von „der" Umwelt im Sinne einer objektiv messbaren Außenwelt der Person die Rede, sondern es wird eben auch parallel dazu die subjektive Sicht der Umwelt berücksichtigt. Darüber hinaus wird eine Untergliederung des Umweltbegriffs in *nahe* und *distante Umwelt*, in *Mikro-Umwelt* (Lebensbereiche), *Meso-Umwelt* (Gemeinde) und *Makro-Umwelt* (Gesellschaft) vorgenommen. Auch ist bei der ökologischen Perspektive eine Differenzierung in *Lebensbereiche* (Arbeit, Wohnen, Familie usw.) und *Dimensionen* wie *physisch-materielle* und *ideell-informatorische Dimension* usw. üblich (Bronfenbrenner 1979; Tretter 2008; Tretter & Löffler-Stastka 2019). Wenngleich diese begriffliche Taxonomie, wie sie vor allem von Uri Bronfenbrenner ausgearbeitet wurde, für die hier zu diskutierende Sinn-Thematik teilweise überbestimmt ist, erlaubt sie auch, einiges an unklaren umweltbezogenen Diskussionen zu spezifizieren, worin auch ihr wissenschaftlicher Wert besteht.

Es können also vorläufig zusammenfassend wenigstens drei vertikal verknüpfte Sinnebenen mit jeweils einer horizontalen Dimension, die von der Person ausgeht, unterschieden werden.

1. Einzelne *punktuelle Erfahrungen*, die in einem Zusammenhang eines fokalen Geschehens erlebt werden, und die Dissonanzen erzeugen und zu affektiv-kognitiven Umstrukturierungen veranlassen, um wieder einen sinnhaften Zusammenhang des Erlebens herstellen zu können.
2. Die Beziehungen zur *konkreten Lebenswelt* mit ihren verschiedenen Bereichen wie Arbeit, Familie usw., die zu Sinnkrisen führen können, etwa durch den

Verlust eines zentralen Teils der Lebenswelt wie der Arbeit, des Lebenspartners oder Wohnung und mit dem damit verbundenen Verlust der Orientierung und damit des Lebenssinns.
3. Die Grunderfahrung der Existenz, mit dem Erleben der Geworfenheit, des In-der-Welt-Seins, der Situiertheit, also umformuliert: die *erlebte Beziehung der Person zu ihrer Umwelt*, oder „Ich und die Welt“, mit der Frage: „Was soll ich tun, was ist mir aufgegeben?“

Anzumerken wäre hier noch, dass in der Humanökologie als Erforschung der Mensch-Umwelt-Beziehungen nicht nur die Umwelt differenziert gesehen wird, sondern auch die *Person* (Tretter 2008): sie wird grundlegend als *bio-psycho-soziales Wesen* im Sinne von Engel verstanden (Engel 1977). Mit den humanökologischen begrifflichen Differenzierungen, die auch wieder aufeinander bezogen sind, wird der dadurch diversifizierte Gesamtsachverhalt der Mensch-Umwelt-Beziehungen allerdings bereits sehr komplex. Um hier wieder mehr analytische Transparenz zu schaffen, wird die *Systemperspektive* vorgeschlagen, die theoriestrategisch durch ihre mathematische Orientierung präzisere konzeptuelle Differenzierungen, Verknüpfungen und Orientierungen ermöglicht als dies rein verbal formulierte Konzepte bieten. In diesem Text wird auf die konzeptuelle Differenzierung der Innenperspektive fokussiert.

Die systemwissenschaftliche Perspektive – Begriffe, Methoden und Modelle

Die *Systemwissenschaft* umfasst heutzutage nicht nur die interdisziplinär verwendeten *Systemtheorien*, die sich auf paradigmatische empirische Beispiele stützen (Bertalanffy 1968; Haken 1977), sondern auch diejenigen Bereiche, die spezifische, aber „supradisziplinär“ verwendete *Begriffe* wie *System*, *Netzwerk*, *Gleichgewicht* usw. umfassen und vor allem die Entwicklung typischer *Methoden* der Systemanalyse und Modellierung ausmachen (Mobus & Kalton 2015). Der Hauptentwicklungs- und Anwendungsbereich der Systemwissenschaft liegt in der Physik und Chemie, in den letzten Jahren kamen die Biologie (Noble 2006b), die Medizin (Tretter 2005), die Psychologie (Schiepek et al. 2015; Tschacher et al. 1992; Kriz 1999; Tretter & Löffler-Stastka 2018) und auch die Soziologie (Luhmann 1984) hinzu. Allerdings ist hier anzumerken, dass die Anwendungen von Systemtheorien in den Sozial-, Geistes- und Verhaltenswissenschaften stark metaphorisch einzustufen sind, insofern zwar qualitativ betrachtet bei sozialen Systemen Ähnlichkeiten zu physikochemischen Systemen gefunden werden können, aber die messtheoretischen Voraussetzungen, beispielsweise was die Interpretation der Variablen, Koeffizientenschätzungen usw. angeht, nicht gegeben sind, vor allem wenn es um *quantitative Modellierungen* und *Computersimulationen* geht. Diese Einschränkungen betreffen auch die folgenden Abschnitte dieses Textes.

Besonders typisch für die systemwissenschaftliche Analyse ist die *Methodik* des Managements von *Zusammenhängen in Theorie und Praxis:* in der Systemwissenschaft geht man methodisch nämlich grundlegend so vor, dass interdisziplinär bzw. transdisziplinär (Forschung und Praxis) ein *integriertes Zooming-in und Zooming-out,* also eine explizite *De-Kontextualisierung* durch die Binnenanalyse des Systems (ggfs. bis zu den Molekülen) und verbunden damit eine *Re-Kontextualisierung* (bis zu den gesellschaftlichen Rahmenbedingungen eines Phänomens) vorgenommen wird. Daraus ergeben sich *Mehr-Ebenen-Systemmodelle*, die auch auf unterschiedlichen Theoremen (z. B. dem Gleichgewichtstheorem) aufbauen. Als besonderes Merkmal gelten schließlich computergestützte explorative Systemmodellierungen u. -analysen. Formaler Hintergrund dafür sind für qualitative und quantitative *Analysen von Strukturen* die Korrelationsanalyse und die Graphentheorie und zur *Analyse von Dynamiken* Differential-Gleichungen, Markov-Ketten usw. Sie stützen sich auf theoretische Paradigmen wie jene der Theorie der dynamischen Systeme, Theorie der nichtlinearen Systeme, Theorien der Selbstorganisation, Netzwerktheorien und Regelungstheorien.

Im Folgenden werden einzelne Aspekte herausgegriffen, um einige systemische Interpretationen des Sinn-Phänomens zu veranschaulichen.

Sinnhafte Netzwerke und das affektiv-kognitive Schema

Hier wird grundlegend davon ausgegangen, dass „Sinn“ erlebt wird, wenn die Erfahrung einer *konsistenten bzw. kohärenten Beziehung* der Person zu einem Erlebnisobjekt als Teil eines umfassenderen Systems gemacht wird, also der Bezug zu einem größeren Ganzen bzw. übergreifenden Werten ohne gravierende Bruchstellen erfahren wird. Es handelt sich also um *Ordnungsgrade* der erlebten äußeren Welt, bezogen auf die Person, und zwar in Form der inneren affektiv-kognitiven Schemata. Bei diesem Modell spielt das Konzept vom personalen *Selbst* eine zentrale Rolle (Pauen 2004). Bemerkenswert in diesem Zusammenhang ist, dass auch der soziologische Systemtheoretiker Niklas Luhmann in dem Sinnbegriff eine *Ordnungsform menschlichen Erlebens* gesehen und ihm damit eine systemübergreifende Bedeutung – zwischen sozialem System und psychischen System – eingeräumt hat (Luhmann 1984; s. auch Frick i.d. Band): Nach

Luhmann differenziert Sinn die Möglichkeiten und Nicht-Möglichkeiten und reduziert Komplexität, die er aber auch zugleich steigert, und zwar durch den Anschluss zu neuen Möglichkeiten. Diese funktionale Charakterisierung passt gut zu der hier im Folgenden für analytische Zwecke dargestellten Netzwerk-Konzeption.

Ein „Netzwerk" kann wie ein „System" mengentheoretisch orientiert als die *Menge von Elementen und ihren Relationen* verstanden werden (Hall & Fagen 1956). Zu beachten ist hier allerdings, dass – genau genommen – ein Netzwerk, im Gegensatz zu einem System, keine konstitutive *Grenzstruktur* hat, denn der Rand des Netzwerks „verläuft" sich gewissermaßen in den Randelementen, die nicht miteinander verbunden sind.

Elemente von Netzwerken (und Systemen) haben unterschiedlich viele Verbindungen untereinander, manche haben eine *zentrale Position* und so führt eine Aktivität bzw. Aktivierung dieses Elements zu einer Aktivierung vieler weiterer Elemente, während eher randständige Elemente, wenn sie aktiviert werden, nur wenige andere Elemente aktivieren.

Die theoretisch-formale Beschreibung und Analyse der Untersuchung der funktionellen Struktur von Netzwerken kann mithilfe der *Graphentheorie* erfolgen, deren formale Wurzeln bis zu dem genialen Mathematiker Leonhard Euler (1707–1783) zurückreichen, die aber neuerdings wieder in der Psychopathologie zur Syndromanalyse genutzt wird (Tretter 2013; Borsboom 2017; Contreras et al 2019).

Folgende Aspekte determinieren die Dynamik eines Netzwerks: die „Zentralität" eines Elements, sie gibt die Position des Elements im Netzwerk an, der „Grad" des Elements der dessen Zahl der Verbindungen angibt und die „Konnektivität" des Netzwerks, die den allgemeinen Grad der Verbindungen im Netzwerk charakterisiert (Diestel 2017). Es werden auch *stabile Graphen* und *instabile Graphen* unterschieden, je nachdem, ob eine *gerade Anzahl* von „negativen" (z. B. hemmenden) Beziehungen oder eine *ungerade Anzahl* derselben vorliegt. Stabile Graphen werden auch als *balancierte Graphen* bezeichnet, sie ergeben eine *konsistente Konfiguration*, während instabile Graphen als *unbalancierte Graphen* bezeichnet werden, die eine *inkonsistente Konfiguration* darstellen. Einfache Strukturen – Dyaden, Triaden, Tetraden usw. – werden als Referenzmodule verwendet, um auch komplexere Graphen auf ihre Stabilitätseigenschaften hin zu untersuchen. Dies erfolgt computerisiert auf der Basis von graphentheoretischen Algorithmen (Alon 2007), was hier nur skizziert wird.

Theorie der kognitiven Dissonanzen und Sinn als Konsistenz

Systemmathematische Grundgedanken, wie jene der Topologie, Vektorrechnung und Graphentheorie, hatten in der Psychologie als Präzisierungen der Gestalt- und Feldtheorie von Kurt Lewin bereits Mitte des 20. Jahrhundert etwa im Rahmen der sogenannten *Konsistenz-Theorien* Eingang gefunden (Heider 1946; Cartwright & Harari 1956; Festinger 1957; Osgood & Tannenbaum 1955). In Fortsetzung dieser Forschungsrichtung kann man davon ausgehen, dass Erfahrungen abgegrenzt, aber verbunden sind, teilweise Abbildungen der Außenwelt und teilweise Konstrukte des Geistigen sind und darüber hinaus affektiv „geladen" sind. Auf diese Weise ergibt sich dann ein Bild von der Welt in Form eines hochgradig detaillierten Netzwerks, das in der Psychologie häufig in Anlehnung an Jean Piaget als *affektiv-kognitives Schema* bezeichnet wird (Piaget 1981; Beck & Alford 1997). Diese Schemata, so die Hypothese, sind Gefüge von kognitiven Elementen mit unterschiedlicher affektiver „Ladung", die grundlegend Elemente des Selbstbilds und Repräsentationen relevanter Umfeldelemente (z. B. Bezugspersonen) umfassen.

Unabhängig von dem Auf und Ab dieser Forschungsrichtung in der Psychologiegeschichte haben sich heute in der klinischen Psychologie zur Charakterisierung des Ordnungsgrades der affektiv-kognitiven Strukturen ähnliche Begriffe in einem strukturorientierten Begriffsverständnis etabliert, wobei vor allem die Begriffe des klinischen Systempsychologen Klaus Grawe und seines Kollegen Franz Caspar genutzt wurde (Grawe 2004a; Caspar 2002): „*Konsistenz*" als Bezeichnung der Schlüssigkeit der kognitiven Repräsentationen, vor allem auf semantischer Ebene, „*Kohärenz*" im dynamischen Vollzug affektiv-kognitiver Prozesse, also in der Erlebnisverarbeitung, und „*Konkordanz*" zur Kennzeichnung der Stimmigkeit des inneren Bedürfnisgefüges. „*Kongruenz*" als Passung disparater Erlebnisinhalte wäre ein weiterer Begriff zur Strukturqualität affektiv-kognitiver Strukturen.

Sie dienen gewissermaßen dazu, die „gute" bzw. „ungute" Gestalt affektiv-kognitiver Schemata und Prozesse zu charakterisieren, und sind somit Ausdrücke für deren *Strukturqualität*. Anzumerken ist hier auch die partielle Korrespondenz mit dem Modell des *Kohärenzsinns*, das Aron Antonovsky zum Verständnis salutogenetischer Prozesse entwickelt hat (Antonovsky 1997).

Inkonsistenz von Rauchen und Gesundheit

Als didaktisch eingängiges *Beispiel* zur Strukturdynamik kognitiver Schemata kann das instabile kognitive Schema dienen, dass Rauchen zwar angenehm erlebt wird, aber mit einem Krebsrisiko verbunden ist: diese *inkonsistente bzw. instabile Konstellation* affektiv-kognitiver Elemente kann durch das Einführen des Gedankens, dass die Person (also „Ich“) *jederzeit mit dem Rauchen aufhören* kann, in eine *stabile Konstellation* übergeführt werden, die das Weiterrauchen affektiv-kognitiv erlaubt: aus *einer negativen Wirkungsrelation*, die auf die Person gerichtet ist und die kennzeichnend für eine *instabile Konfiguration* ist, werden *zwei negative Relationen* und damit eine *stabile Konfiguration* erreicht (Abb. 3). Man kann nun sagen, dass die Person nach der Einsicht in den „Unsinn“ des Rauchens wieder „sinnhaft“ rauchen kann, wenngleich dies aus realistischen Gründen ein Selbstbetrug ist, denn Rauchen macht süchtig und das Risiko nimmt objektiv mit der Zeit zu usw. Diese weiteren Relationen seien hier aber nur erwähnt.

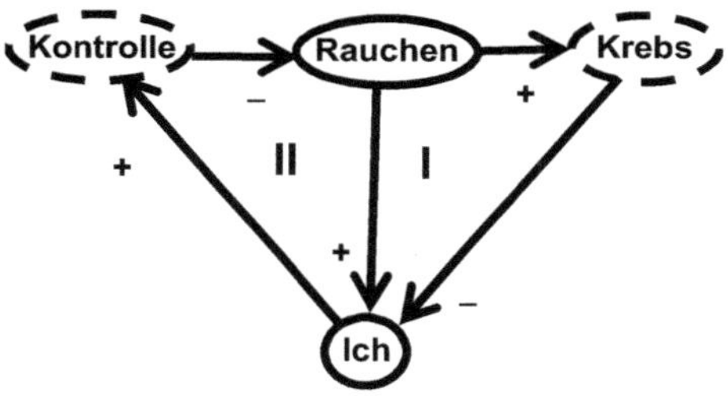

Abb. 3: Für die Person (Ich) angenehmes Rauchen (+), mit dem unangenehmen Risiko, Krebs zu bekommen (*eine* negative Relation, I), und die *Balancierung* durch den Gedanken, jederzeit mit dem Rauchen aufhören zu können (*zweite* negative Relation, II).

Die Bedeutung derartiger Restrukturierungsprozesse hat Grawe als Basisprinzip der psychischen Homöostase angesehen: „...Konsistenzregulation findet ganz überwiegend unbewusst statt und durchzieht so sehr das ganze psychische Geschehen, dass es angemessen erscheint, von einem obersten oder pervasiven Regulationsprinzip im psychischen Geschehen zu sprechen.“ (Grawe 2004b: 190 – 191).

Synergetik als Heuristik für die Dynamik der Sinnfindung

Ein zentraler Begriff, welcher die Verlaufsstrukturen von Prozessen im Zustandsraum, also Zustands-Dynamiken, charakterisiert, ist der Begriff „Gleichgewicht“ (besser: Fließgleichgewicht). Dieser Begriff impliziert den Begriff von „Gewichten“, also von gegenläufigen Kräften, die gewissermaßen – so die Annahme hier – über die Zeit hin fluktuieren bzw. schwingen: *Agonisten* und *Antagonisten* eines Prozesses oder Zustands halten sich gewissermaßen „pendelnd die Waage“. Systeme können *bistabil* (auch multistabil) sein, insofern sie zwei oder mehrere stabile Gleichgewichtszustände aufweisen, wie beispielsweise gesund und auch manchmal krank zu sein. Diese Gleichgewichtsbereiche werden auch heute im Kontext von Theorien nichtlinearer Systeme als *Attraktoren* der Zustandsverläufe bezeichnet, während Hindernisse, Schwellen oder Rückstellkräfte als *Repelloren* bezeichnet werden. Ein Kernbereich der Systemtheorien ist dann die *Analyse von Dynamiken* mit nichtlinearem, ja sprunghaftem Verlauf oder polymorphem Verlauf, bei dem glatte und sprunghafte Zustandsänderungen auftreten können (Katastrophentheorie, Chaostheorie; Tretter 2005).

Ein bewährtes Beispiel für solche formalen Ansätze ist die *Synergetik* von Hermann Haken (Haken 1977): die variierende Dynamik des Systems lässt sich aus dem Wirken von einem energetisierenden *Kontrollparameter* und einem strukturbildenden *Ordnungsparameter* herleiten. Für unsere Fragestellung der Bedingungen der *Sinnfindung* wäre also der Ordnungsparameter gewissermaßen die Strukturqualität des affektiv-kognitiven semantischen Netzwerks und damit ein hypothetischer Faktor für die Sinnfindung, insbesondere bei Übergängen von einer inkonsistenten Sinnstruktur (störendes Ereignis) zu einer Neuordnung: bei einer hohen Aktivierung durch den energetisierenden Kontrollparameter kann die Schwelle, die durch das Repellor-Gebirge gegeben ist, nach einigen kritischen Fluktuationen überwunden werden und eine Neuformation der semantischen Matrix gefunden werden (Abb. 4). Dieses Modell zeigt Ähnlichkeiten mit dem vorher besprochenen Konzept des Lebensraums von Kurt Lewin und auch mit der „Strukturdynamik“ von Werner Janzarik.

Das Regelkreismodell und der Wille zum Sinn

Ein Regelkreis ist ein Modell eines Funktionsgefüges, bei dem ein *Operator* (Effektor, Aktuator) über einen *Sensor* und einen *Regulator* kreisförmig zusammen-

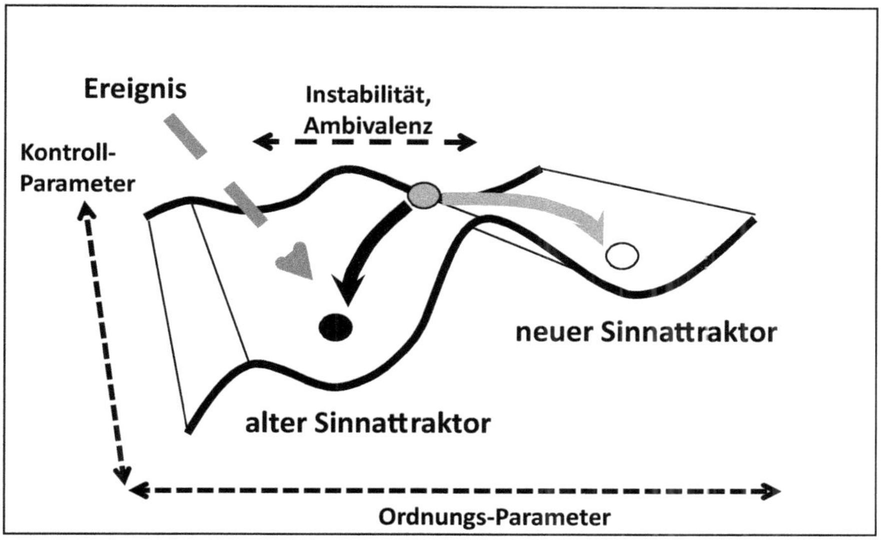

Abb. 4: Die Potenziallandschaft der Synergetik. Der Kontrollparameter prägt die Gestalt der Landschaft, mit ihren Tälern der Stabilität (Attraktoren) und den hinderlichen Gebirgen (Repelloren), die als Grenzbereiche mit instabilem Verhalten (Ambivalenz) Optionen für Rückbildungen oder Neubildungen der Systemzustände bieten. Der Kontrollparameter führt dazu, dass sich das System (Kugel im Bild) in verschiedene Zustandsbereiche (z. B. linkes Tal oder rechtes Tal) bewegt und dort verweilt (Attraktor-Effekt) oder hin und her fluktuiert (instabiler Bereich).

geschaltet ist, und das gemäß einer Diskrepanz von gespeicherten *Sollwerten* und registrierten *Istwerten* operiert.

Dieses Modell korrespondiert mit dem Konzept von Frankl, das mit dem „Willen zum Sinn“ beschrieben wird und vor allem als Abgrenzung von dem triebmechanischen Modell von Sigmund Freud als zentraler Antrieb des Menschen angesehen werden kann. Viktor Frankl sagte (Frankl 2006: 155): „Es ist keine Schande sein Ziel nicht zu erreichen, aber es ist eine Schande kein Ziel zu haben!“ Führt man diesen Gedanken weiter aus, so ergibt sich folgendes Bild: „Da es dem Menschen in seinem Willen zum Sinn nicht um ein inneres Gleichgewicht geht, sondern um Sinn und Werte an sich, entsteht „eine ständige Spannung zwischen Sein und Sollen“ („Noodynamik“; Spektrum 2020). Dieser Aspekt des Konzepts „Wille zum Sinn“ lässt sich in das Bild einer Istwert-Sollwert-Diskrepanz transponieren und zum kybernetischen *Regelkreismodell* erweitern (Abb. 5), das auch dem *Funktionskreismodell* des Biologen Jakob von Uexküll entspricht, das die Lebewesen-Umwelt-Interaktion modellieren soll (Uexküll 1909). Es korrespondiert in ähnlicher Weise mit dem bewährten *handlungstheoretischen Pha-*

senmodell von Willensprozessen des Psychologen Heinz Heckhausen („Rubikon-Modell“; Heckhausen u. Heckhausen 2010) und es ist auch verknüpft mit der phänomenologischen Sicht (Fuchs 2016): bei jeder Willensbildung tritt ein Stadium ein, bei dem die zunächst ambivalente oder polyvalente innere Situation der Motive, Vorstellungen usw. *konsistent* (und *kohärent*) wird und zur Entscheidung führt (Rubikon-Schwelle) und somit „Sinn macht“ für den Handlungsvollzug, dessen Ergebnisse (Istwerte) wieder rückgekoppelt werden, und zwar mit den mit dem Willensprozess verknüpften Erwartungen (Sollwerten). Der Willensprozess macht das Ziel zum Sinn, d. h. der Sinn als Kohärenz der Motive ermöglicht die Formation des Willens als Handlungsplan. Der Grad der Kongruenz von Soll und Ist ergibt auch die Gefühlslage: Freude und Lust bei hoher Kongruenz, bei niedriger Kongruenz Ärger, Angst oder gar Gedrücktheit, Trauer, Depression. Die Gefühlslage aktiviert wiederum verschiedene Motive (z. B. das Bedürfnis nach sozialer Anerkennung) und ein weiterer Handlungszyklus wird realisiert usw. (Abb. 5)

Dieses Regelkreismodell menschlichen Handelns, das an anderer Stelle detaillierter ausgearbeitet wurde (Tretter & Löffler-Stastka 2018), mag mechanistisch erscheinen, es eignet sich aber gut als Heuristik in der Therapie, und zwar nicht nur für den Therapeuten, sondern auch für die Klienten (Tretter & Müller 2001).

Folgerungen

Der Begriff „Sinn“ zeigt eine semantische Vielfalt mit unzähligen Unschärfen, welche die interdisziplinäre wissenschaftliche Erforschung und das Verstehen von „Sinn“ erschweren. Sinn steht – wenngleich er lebenspraktisch und therapeutisch äußerst wichtig ist – in psychologischer Sicht singulär zu gängigen theoretischen Konzepten und müsste daher stärker in ein Gesamtverständnis bzw. in ein integratives Modell psychischer Prozesse eingefügt werden. Der bekannte „Schulenstreit“, der oft pragmatisch mit dem Begriff „Polypragmasie“ nivelliert wird, ohne dass theoretische Integrationskonzepte vorliegen, kann – wie hier vorgeschlagen wird – durch eine *humanökologische Rahmenkonzeption* und eine *systemische Konzeption* des Psychischen theoretisch überbrückt werden. Der theoretische Vorteil der ökologischen Perspektive ist die Grundannahme der Situiertheit des Menschen und damit die Abhängigkeit des Sinnerlebens von der externen Situation, wobei dieses aber auch innerpsychisch durch *Gleichgewichte (bzw. Paritäten), Konsistenzen, Kongruenzen* und *Kohärenzen* affektiv-kognitiver Strukturen determiniert ist. Bei der formalen Explikation des Strukturellen und der Dynamik des Phänomens Sinn im psychischen Bereich kann die Systemtheorie zu konzeptionellen Präzisierungen verhelfen. Sinn wird in dieser Hinsicht

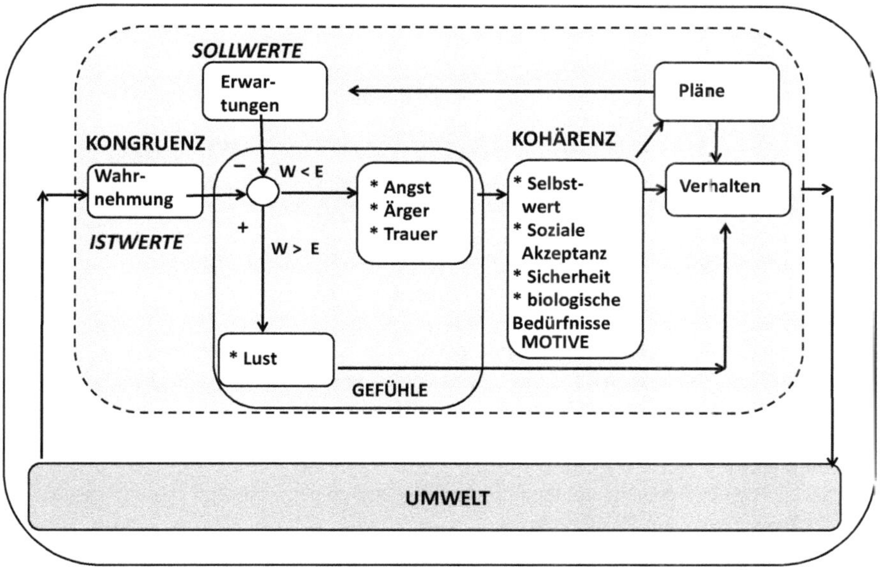

Abb. 5: Die funktionelle Struktur der Psyche als Regelkreis zwischen Person und Umwelt. Die Kohärenz von *Motiven*, die Entscheidungen zur *Handlungsplanung* erst ermöglicht, treibt das zielgerichtete *Verhalten* (Handeln) an, mit dem Ergebnis, dass beispielsweise Umweltveränderungen bewirkt werden, die *wahrgenommen* werden und mit den *Ergebnis- Erwartungen* verknüpft werden. Bei Kongruenzen tritt Erleben von „sinnhaftem Handeln“ ein, mit entsprechenden angenehmen Gefühlen, bei Inkongruenzen treten negative Gefühle auf, die wiederum eine neue Motivdynamik zur Folge haben können, mit der Folge neuer Handlungspläne usw. (Q: veränd. nach Tretter & Löffler-Stastka 2017)

grundlegend als *Strukturqualität* der affektiv-kognitiven Schemata angesehen und auf diese Weise mit traditionsreichen theoretischen Konzepten der Psychologie in Verbindung gebracht. Dabei kann die *Graphentheorie* zur Strukturanalyse nützen, und die Synergetik kann die *Sinndynamik* als Wirkung eines *Attraktors* verdeutlichen, in den mehrere verschiedene Initialzustände „hineinlaufen“. Auch erscheint ein Regelkreismodell, das die Diskrepanz von Sollwert und Istwert als Vitalisierungsbedingung des Mentalen ansieht, in Hinblick auf den „Willen zum Sinn“ nützlich.

Einige Bausteine für derartige Modellier-Projekt wurden hier skizzenhaft vorgestellt. Sie müssten unter Bezug auf den Ansatz von Viktor Frankl im interdisziplinären Kontext weiter diskutiert werden und in einem nächsten Schritt detaillierter und an konkreten Anwendungsbeispielen geprüft werden.

Literatur

Alon U (2007) An introduction to systems biology: design principles of biological circuits. Boca Raton: Chapman & Hall.

Antonovsky A (1997) Salutogenese. Zur Entmystifizierung der Gesundheit. Tübingen: dgvt.

Barker RG (1968) Ecological Psychology: Concepts and Methods for Studying the Environment of Human Behavior. Palo Alto, CA: Stanford University Press.

Beck AT, Alford BA (1997) The Integrative Power of Cognitive Therapy. New York, London: Guilford Press.

Bertalanffy L (1968) General system theory: Foundations, Development. New York, NY: George Braziller.

Borsboom D (2017). A network theory of mental disorders. In: World Psychiatry 16: 5–13.

Bourdieu P (2004) Das Paradox des Soziologen. In: Bourdieu, Pierre (Hg.): Soziologische Fragen. Frankfurt am Main: Suhrkamp. 83–91.

Bronfenbrenner U (1979) The Ecology of Human Development. Cambridge, MA: Harvard University Press.

Brunswik E (1956) Perception and the representative design of psychological experiments. Berkeley: University of California Press.

Cartwright D, Harary F (1956) Structural balance: a generalization of Heider's theory. In: Psychol. Rev. 63:277–293.

Caspar F (2002) Ätiologie und Therapie psychischer Störungen aus der Sicht eines integrativen Modelles. In: Ahrens S, Schneider W (Hg.) Lehrbuch der Psychotherapie und Psychosomatischen Medizin. Stuttgart/ New York: Schattauer. 569–580.

Contreras A, Nieto I, Valiente C, Espinosa R, Vazquez C (2019) The Study of Psychopathology from the Network Analysis Perspective: A Systematic Review. Psychother Psychosom 88:71–83.

Diestel R (2017) Graphentheorie. Berlin: Springer.

Engel GL (1977) The need for a new medical model: a challenge for biomedicine. In: Science 196(4286): 129–136.

Festinger L (1957) A Theory of Cognitive Dissonance. Stanford, CA: Row, Peterson.

Frankl VE (1994) Die Sinnfrage in der Psychotherapie. München.

Frankl VE (1997a) Der Wille zum Sinn. Ausgewählte Vorträge über Logotherapie. München.

Frankl VE (1997b) Das Leiden am sinnlosen Leben. Psychotherapie für heute. Freiburg, Basel, Wien.

Frankl VE (2006) Der Mensch vor der Frage nach dem Sinn. Eine Auswahl aus dem Gesamtwerk. 19. Auflage. München: Piper.

Fuchs T (2016) Wollen können. Wille, Selbstbestimmung und psychische Krankheit. In: Moos T, Rehmann-Sutter C, Schües C (Hg) Randzonen des Willens. Anthropologische und ethische Probleme von Entscheidungen in Grenzsituationen. Praktische Philosophie kontrovers. Frankfurt am Main: Peter Lang.

Gibson JJY (1977) The theory of affordances. In: Shaw RE, Bransford J (Hg.) Perceiving, Acting and Knowing. Milton Park: Taylor & Francis Group.

Glaeser B (1989) Humanoekologie. Opladen: Westdeutscher Verlag.

Glaeser B, Teherani-Krönner P (1992) Humanökologie und Kulturökologie. Opladen: Westdeutscher Verlag.

Glasersfeld E (1996) Der Radikale Konstruktivismus. Ideen, Ergebnisse, Probleme. Frankfurt a. M.: Suhrkamp.
Grawe K (2004a) Psychological Therapy. Ashland, OH: Hogrefe & Huber Publishers.
Grawe K (2004b) Neuropsychotherapie. Hogrefe: Göttingen.
Haeckel E (1866) Generelle Morphologie der Organismen. Berlin: Reimer.
Haken H (1977) Synergetics. New York, NY: Springer.
Hall AD, Fagen RE (1956). Definition of system. In: Gen. Syst. 1:18–28.
Heckhausen J, Heckhausen H (2010) Motivation and Action. Cambridge: Cambridge University Press.
Heider F (1946) Attitudes and Cognitive Organization. In: Journal of Psychology 21:107–112.
Janzarik W (1988). Strukturdynamische Grundlagen der Psychiatrie. Jena: Enke.
Kinast G, Fischer M (1999) Existenzanalyse und Logotherapie. Linz.
Knötig H (Hg.) (1976) Proceedings of the First International Meeting on Human Ecology, Vienna 1975. St. Saphorin: Georgi.
Knötig H (Hg.) (1979) Proceedings of the Second International Meeting on Human Ecology, Vienna 1977. St.Saphorin: Georgi.
Kriz J (1999) Systemtheorie für Psychotherapeuten, Psychologen und Mediziner: Eine Einführung. Wien: Facultas.
Längle A (1988) Entscheidung zum Sein. Viktor Frankls Logotherapie in der Praxis. München: Piper.
Längle A (2005) Das Sinnkonzept V. Frankls – ein Beitrag für die gesamte Psychotherapie. In: Petzold HG, Orth I (Hg.) Sinn, Sinnerfahrung, Lebenssinn in Psychologie und Psychotherapie. Bd. II. Bielefeld/Locarno: Aisthesis. 403–460.
Lampersberger F (2014) Eine philosophische Untersuchung des Sinnbegriffs. In: Logotherapie und Existenzanalyse von Viktor Frankl. Saarbrücken: Akademikerverlag.
Lewin K, Heider F, Heider GM (1936) Principles of Topological Psychology. New York, NY: McGraw-Hill Book Company.
Lewin K (1951) Field Theory in Social Science: Selected Theoretical Papers. Oxford: Harper.
Luhmann N (1984) Soziale Systeme. Grundriß einer allgemeinen Theorie. Frankfurt: Suhrkamp.
Maturana HR, Varela FJ (1987) Der Baum der Erkenntnis. Die biologischen Wurzeln menschlichen Erkennens. Bern, München, Wien: Scherz.
Mobus GE, Kalton MC (2015). Principles of Systems Science. New York, NY: Springer.
Mühlum A, Olschowy G, Oppl H, Wendt WR (Hg.) (1986) Umwelt? Lebenswelt: Beiträge zu Theorie und Praxis ökosozialer Arbeit. Frankfurt: Diesterweg.
Nagel T (1974) What is it like to be a bat? Philosophical Review. LXXXIII (4): 435–450.
Noble D (2006) Music of Life: Biology beyond genes. Oxford: Oxford Univ. Press.
Park RE, Burgess EW, McKenzie RD (1925) The city. Chicago: University of Chicago Press.
Oppl H, Weber-Falkensammer H (Hg.) (1986): Lebenslagen und Gesundheit. 3 Bde. Frankfurt: Diesterweg.
Osgood CE, Tannenbaum PH (1955) The principle of congruity in the prediction of attitude change. In: Psychological Review, 62(1): 42–55.
Pauen M (2004) Illusion Freiheit? Mögliche oder unmögliche Konsequenzen der Hirnforschung. Frankfurt: Fischer.
Piaget J (1981) Meine Theorie der geistigen Entwicklung. 2. Aufl. 2010. Weinheim, Basel: Beltz.
Psillos S (1999) Scientific Realism: How Science tracks Truth, New York and London: Routledge.

Schiepek G, Eckert H, Aas B, Wallot S, Wallot A (2015) Integrative Psychotherapy: A Feedback-Driven Dynamic Systems Approach. Boston, MA: Hogrefe Publishing.
Schütz A, Luckmann T (1975) Strukturen der Lebenswelt. Luchterhand, Neuwied
Serbser WH (2004) Humanökologie. München: Oekom.
Thiersch H (2015) Soziale Arbeit und Lebensweltorientierung. Gesammelte Aufsätze. Weinheim, Basel.
Spektrum (2020) Lexikon der Psychologie – Wille zum Sinn. https://www.spektrum.de/lexikon/psychologie/wille-zum-sinn/16850.
Tretter F, Müller A (2001) Psychologische Therapie der Sucht. Göttingen: Hogrefe.
Tretter F (2005) Systemtheorie im klinischen Kontext. Lengerich: Pabst.
Tretter F (2008) Ökologie der Person. Lengerich: Pabst.
Tretter F (2013) Systemtheorie des Wahns – graphentheoretische Perspektiven. In: Stompe T (Hg) Wahnalysen. Berlin: Med.Wiss. Verlag. 33–50.
Tretter F, Löffler-Stastka H (2018) Steps Toward an Integrative Clinical Systems Psychology. In: Front. Psychol. 9:1616.
Tretter F, Löffler-Stastka H (2019) The Human Ecological Perspective and Biopsychosocial Medicine. Int J Environ Res Public Health 6(21):4230.
Tschacher W, Schiepek G, Brunner EJ (1992) Self-Organization and Clinical Psychology. Berlin: Springer.
Uexküll J (1909) Umwelt und Innenwelt der Tiere Berlin: Springer.
Wallner F (1992) Acht Vorlesungen über den Konstruktiven Realismus. Wien: Wiener Universitäts-Verlag.
Watzlawick P (1976) Wie wirklich ist die Wirklichkeit – Wahn, Täuschung, Verstehen. München: Piper.

Ralf T. Vogel

Der Dunkle Sinn

Die Sinnfrage im Kontext des Schattenkonzepts der Analytischen Psychologie

Dark Meaning
The question of meaning in the context of the 'shadow-concept' in Analytical Psychology

Zusammenfassung: Die Konzeptionen von Sinn und Sinnerfahrung werden in Philosophie und (Tiefen-)Psychologie oft unhinterfragt positiviert und moralisch als wertvoll deklariert. Die Schattenkonzeption der Analytischen Psychologie und die durch sie inspirierte bipolare Sinnauffassung zeigt auf, dass auch mit einer dunklen Seite des Sinns zu rechnen ist, die etwa in raschen Sinnzuschreibungen an negative Ereignisse wie Leid und Krise oder aber auch durch Sinnerleben in negativ-destruktiven Handlungen in Erscheinung tritt. Die notwendige Konsequenz ist eine beständige Bewusstmachung dieser dunklen Sinnseiten in jedem Einzelnen und eine verantwortete Positionierung dazu.

Schlüsselwörter: Schattenkonzept, C.G. Jung, Analytische Psychologie

Abstract: The conceptions of meaning and the experience of meaningfulness are predominately presented positively in philosophy as well as in (depth-)psychology, and are mostly declared as morally valuable. The shadow conception of C.G. Jung's Analytical Psychology and the bipolar conception of meaning inspired by it show that a dark side of meaning has to be taken into consideration. This dark side appears, for example, in rapid attributions of meaning to negative events such as suffering and crisis, or in the experiences of meaningfulness in negative and destructive acts. The necessary consequence is a constant effort to heighten awareness of these dark sides of meaning in oneself, and to position oneself responsibly in relation to them.

Keywords: Shadow Concept, C.G. Jung, Analytical Psychology

Der Ausgangpunkt

Das psychologische Denkgebäude, von dem der vorliegende Beitrag seinen Ausgang nimmt, ist die Analytische Psychologie. Da diese evtl. nicht jedem/jeder

https://doi.org/10.1515/9783110787153-009

Leser/-in vertraut ist, hier ein paar wenige Vorbemerkungen. Unter den Terminus der Analytischen Psychologie fasst man einen (tiefen-)psychologischen Theorie- und Methodenkanon, der von dem Schweizer Psychiater und Psychologen C.G. Jung (1856 – 1961) begründet und seitdem international fortwährend weiterentwickelt wurde. Auch als Jung'sche Psychologie oder Psychoanalyse nach C.G. Jung bezeichnet, hat sie bis heute einen deutlichen Bezug zu ihrem Gründervater, dessen Schriften allerdings nicht mehr als die abschließende Autorität, jedoch immer noch als Startpunkt der Denkentwicklungen gilt. Jung gab seiner Psychologie eine deutliche Zuordnung auf den Weg. War er zunächst als Arzt und gar Experimentalpsychologe naturwissenschaftlichen und messenden Methoden der psychologischen Erkenntnisgewinnung durchaus zugeneigt, so änderte sich dies im Laufe seiner Entwicklung, spätestens aber nach seinen dramatischen inneren Erlebnissen zwischen den Jahren 1914 und 1918 rasch und durchaus radikal in Richtung sozial-, kultur- und geisteswissenschaftlicher Topoi und auch Methoden sowie in Richtung einer zumindest partiellen Zuordnung seiner Psychologie zur Philosophie: „Ich kann es kaum verschleiern, dass wir Psychotherapeuten eigentlich philosophische Ärzte oder ärztliche Philosophen sein sollten, oder vielmehr dass wir es schon sind, ohne es wahr haben zu wollen...“, so Jung 1943 (GW 16: § 181). Schließlich schälte sich eine genuin analytisch-psychologische Erkenntnistheorie heraus, die, in gängigen Termini formuliert, Überschneidungen mit der Phänomenologie, dem (bisweilen sogar Radikalen) Skeptizismus oder der Hermeneutik aufweist, jedoch durchaus eine wissenschaftstheoretische Eigenständigkeit etwa durch die Hervorbringung einer sog. Imaginology einer Wissenschaft vom (inneren) Bild, behaupten kann.

Zur Metapher des Dunklen

Das Dunkle wird in den mitteleuropäischen Kulturen ambivalent betrachtet. Zum einen gibt es das Dunkle in Gestalt des Unsichtbaren, schwer Erkennbaren, Geheimnisvollen. Dunkel bleibt uns die Bedeutung von etwas, wir verstehen es nicht oder nicht ganz und versuchen, ‚Licht in die Sache zu bringen‘. Die von ostasiatischen Spiritualitäten bekannte ‚Erleuchtung‘ steht ebenso in der Tradition dieser Kampfansage an etwas, das (noch) nicht erkannt oder verstanden wurde. Erleuchtung ist aber nicht nur das Ziel buddhistischer Meditation. Auch das Zeitalter der Aufklärung wird bekanntlich im Englischen als ‚enlightenment‘, eben als Erleuchtung bezeichnet, hinein in die Finsternis von Aberglauben und Unwissenheit. Sie ist der Beginn der Skepsis gegenüber dem Unbekannten und Unbewussten, die ab jetzt im Verdacht stehen, schädlich oder gar böse zu sein. Das Dunkle tritt uns mehr und mehr gegenüber in Gestalt des Negativen, Bösen,

Angstmachenden. Die Nacht, bis dahin eine Lebenszeit gleichberechtigt mit dem Tageslicht, wird bedrohlich, die ‚Kreaturen der Nacht', seien es Phantasiegestalten wie Vampire oder nachtaktive Tiere, bei uns an erster Stelle die Wölfe, werden negativ beschrieben und sollen bekämpft, ja vernichtet werden. Gerade hier aber, im Umgang mit der Nacht als Paradebeispiel des Dunklen, zeigt sich die Ambivalenz des Menschen dem Undurchschaubaren gegenüber. Die Nacht bleibt, neben ihren angsteinflößenden Aspekten, auch die Zeit der großen Feste und Events, sie wird zur Zeit der (sexuellen) Lust und vermittelt nicht selten Schutz und Geborgenheit. Diese Ambivalenz, man könnte auch sagen Bipolarität des Phänomens des Dunklen wird uns im vorliegenden Text eine Richtschnur sein, wenn wir zwei Konzepte miteinander in Verbindung bringen, die in der Analytischen Psychologie in der Nachfolge C.G. Jungs einen zentralen Stellenwert einnehmen, nämlich die Schattenpsychologie und die Wertschätzung der Sinnfrage.

Die Analytische Psychologie und das Sinnkonzept

Maßgebliche jungianische Autor/-innen sind sich einig, dass das Sinnkonzept an zentraler Stelle des theoretischen und v. a. auch therapiepraktischen Werkes C.G. Jungs anzusiedeln ist (Jaffé 1983). „Die Neurose kann letztendlich verstanden werden als ein Leiden der Seele, die ihren Sinn nicht gefunden hat" (GW 11: § 497), so C.G. Jung bereits 1939, jedoch legte er keine stringente und in sich geschlossene Sicht auf den Sinnkontext vor. Auch eine Rezeption der Gedanken seines Zeitgenossen Viktor Frankl ist nicht bekannt (wohingegen dieser Jung nebenbei und nicht selten etwas abschätzig zur Kenntnis nahm) (vgl. z. B. Schock 1994).

Es fällt zunächst auf der eher abstrakten Ebene der Theoriebildung eine ‚Mehrfachnutzung' des Sinnbegriffes bei Jung auf: Erstens finden wir veritable philosophische Überlegungen zur Sinnfrage: Sinn und Lebenssinn werden zu einer metaphysischen Größe, über die spekuliert werden kann. Hier wird ‚Sinn' oft verstanden als Bedeutung oder Bedeutsamkeit. Zweitens, und dies kann durchaus als ein Schwerpunkt Jungs im Sinnkontext gesehen werden, ist Sinn, dessen Fehlen und dessen (Wieder-)Herstellung ein zentrales Agens analytisch-psychologischer Therapie und Psychopathologie. Drittens finden wir die Sinnvokabel in hermeneutischer Tradition genutzt. Hier wird der Sinn eines psychischen Ereignisses, etwa eines Symptoms gesucht, der z. B. im Ausdruck einer seelischen Notlage oder in der Wiederherstellung eines psychischen Gleichgewichts liegen kann. Das Ereignis ist dann als ‚sinnvoll' erkennbar, es ‚macht Sinn'.

Schließlich viertens, und das sei hier nur am Rande bemerkt, da für unseren Zusammenhang nicht zentral, entwickelt Jung im Zusammenhang mit dem Synchronizitätsprinzip einen weiteren Sinngedanken, indem er postuliert, nichtkausale Zusammenhänge, sog. „synchronistische Ereignisse", seien „als die Glieder einer sinngemäßen Koinzidenz durch Gleichzeitigkeit und durch den Sinn verbunden…" (GW 8: § 906).

In der Übersicht über Jungs enormes und, z. B. bezogen auf die vorzufindenden Textsorten, sehr heterogenes Gesamtwerk wird auf der pragmatischen Ebene eine implizite Zweiteilung des Sinnbegriffes deutlich, wie wir sie von anderen Denkern ebenfalls kennen. Die schlagwortartig aus der Analytischen Psychologie längst ins Populäre ausgewanderte Dichotomie in eine introvertierte und eine extravertierte Richtung der Lebensenergie, der sog. Libido ist hier zu nennen. Die 'konkretistische' Sinn-Version Jungs sieht diese am Werk in der Beziehung des Menschen nach Außen, zur Welt, zu den Dingen und den Mitmenschen, in Arbeit, Beziehung und Handeln. Diesem Außeninteresse, wenn es um die Suche nach Sinnerlebnissen geht, kann eine Innenausrichtung der Lebensenergie gegenübergestellt werden. Die introvertierte Sinnerfassung geschieht durch den Bezug auf sich selbst, durch die Erfahrung innerer Entwicklungen, durch das Herausbilden von Werten und Normen etc. Sie erfolgt weniger durch Handeln als vielmehr durch Denken und (in-sich-hinein-)Fühlen. Vor allem (aber nicht nur) dadurch, also in der nach innen gerichteten Schau, baut der Mensch, so Jung, zwangsläufig auch seine Beziehung zur Transzendenz aus, da das den Einzelmenschen Überschreitende primär in ihm selbst zu finden sei und diese inneren Erlebnisse lediglich, bisweilen aber durchaus notwendigerweise, angeregt werden durch Außengeschehnisse wie etwa Naturbetrachtungen oder zwischenmenschliche Beziehungen.

„Gehe nicht nach draußen, kehre in dich selbst ein; im inneren Menschen wohnt die Wahrheit" so ein von Jung sehr geschätzter Satz des Augustinus in *De vera religione*. Es gibt neben der psychologischen also auch eine durchaus ‚metaphysisch' zu nennende Sinn-Version bei Jung und deren wiederum psychologischer Ausdruck ist die Idee des Sinns (bzw. des Sinnerlebens) als archetypisches Geschehen. Es ist hier nicht der Ort, um Jungs Archetypenpsychologie zu entfalten (vgl. dazu z. B. Roesler 2016). Es sei nur so viel gesagt: Die Archetypenlehre könnte als die eigentliche ‚Seelenlehre' Jungs angesehen werden (Vogel 2018). Archetypen können im Sinne der Analytischen Psychologie definiert werden als menschheitsimmanente Strukturierungsmotive. Sie sind, und das ist von großer Bedeutung, per se ‚unanschaulich', unterscheiden sich also vom archetypischen Bild, das schon eine Verarbeitung hindurch durch individuelle und kulturelle Schichten bedeutet. Archetypen haben eine ‚numinose' Wirkung. Sie ergreifen uns, ereignen, konstellieren sich. D. h. sie zu erleben ist nicht herstellbar, sondern allenfalls zulassbar. Archetypen, so Jung, sind bipolar, weisen also wie alles Psychische bei genauer Betrachtung immer eine Gegensatzstruktur auf.

Kommen wir zurück zur Sinnfrage: Zum einen finden wir in der Analytischen Psychologie die Idee des Erlebens des Archetypischen als an sich sinnerfüllend, ja die Konstellation eines Archetyps wird gar als ‚sinnstiftend' bezeichnet, in ihm liegt „eine bis dahin für unmöglich gehaltene Sinnerfülltheit" (GW 8: §405). V. a. die Individuation, der Weg des Menschen hin zu seinem eigentlichen Selbst, der nach Jung ebenfalls archetypischen Gesetzen folgt, vermittelt Sinn, so dass umgekehrt das Erleben von Sinnlosigkeit als Folge von Unterbrechung oder Verlassen des Individuationsweges gedeutet wird. Das Selbst ist das im Leben „Angelegte, auf das hin ich mich entwickle" (Riedel 2009: 38), die immer nur als Möglichkeit gegebene Ganzheit der Persönlichkeit, die alle Polaritäten umgreift.

Neben dieser generellen Sinnwirkung des Archetypischen wird von jungianischen Autor/-innen argumentiert, es gäbe auch einen ‚Archetypen des Sinns' per se, nämlich eben das, was wir bereits als Individuationsziel kennengelernt haben und was Jung als das Selbst bezeichnet, eine Begriffsnutzung, die sich von den Selbstdefinitionen etwa der Psychoanalyse oder der akademischen Psychologie fundamental unterscheidet (Vogel 2016): „Das Selbst hat hauptsächlich den Aspekt des Numinosen schlechthin, des letztlich Überlegenen, als Offenbarung des „Sinns des Lebens" oder des göttlichen inneren Seelenzentrums..." (v. Franz 2014: 453). Die Nähe des personalen und weitgehend bewussten Ich zum Selbst ist hier die primäre Quelle der Sinnerfüllung. Für unseren Zusammenhang ist von Bedeutung: Das Selbst als Archetyp der Ganzheit und des Sinns und oft bebildert als der Alte Weise, der Priester oder der Philosoph, weist natürlich, wie alle Archetypen, auch eine bipolare Gegensatzstruktur auf, d. h. in der Ganzheit umfasst es Positives wie Negatives, Gutes wie Böses. Der ‚Ganze Mensch' und damit auch der sinnerfüllte Mensch ist, und darauf weist uns die Analytische Psychologie immer wieder hin, eben nicht der ‚nur-gute' Mensch sondern derjenige, der die „Transzendente Funktion" als Überbrückerin der Gegensätze zu kultivieren vermag.

Der Schatten in der Analytischen Psychologie

Im Konzept des Schattens vereint Jung Niederschläge der persönlichen Biographie (etwa das Verdrängte und Abgewehrte) mit archetypischen Schichten bis hinein in das kollektiv Böse schlechthin, das nicht mehr mit mir als Individuum, sondern nur noch mit mir als Angehöriger des Menschengeschlechtes zu tun hat. Damit wird der Schatten, der „Dunkle Bruder der Menschheit überhaupt" (Neumann 2009: 65), zum Gegensätzlichen, Fremden, Anderen in mir, das immer und überall mitzudenken ist und das fasziniert und abstößt zugleich.

Der Schatten ist der (augenscheinlich) inferiore Anteil des Menschen. Er liegt größtenteils im Unbewussten und wirkt von dort, umfasst aber auch diejenigen unserer Eigenschaften und Handlungsoptionen, gegen die wir uns bewusst entscheiden, die wir immer wieder bewusst zurückweisen. Das Schattenkonzept der Analytischen Psychologie hat strukturelle Ähnlichkeiten mit dem – ebenfalls die Dunkelmetapher nutzenden – physikalischen Konzept der ‚Dunklen Materie'. Wie sie ist der Schatten nicht direkt beobachtbar, sondern zeigt sich in seinen Auswirkungen und stellt ein sinnvolles Konstrukt dar, um etwa Phänomene wie Hass oder Fremdenfeindlichkeit zu erklären. Der Schatten will (von uns und von der Welt) nicht gesehen werden und wird abgewehrt. Neben dem Dunklen in uns umfasst er auch das „ungelebte Leben". Der Schatten ist, so Jung, „kentaurisch" mit dem Menschen verbunden (GW 5: § 678), wir werden ihn niemals los und sind Zeit unseres Lebens vor die Aufgabe gestellt, ihn anzuerkennen und mit ihm zu ringen. Die Bewusstmachung des Schattens und seiner Schichten ist ein maßgeblicher Teil einer wörtlich gemeinten Selbst-Erkenntnis und darauffolgender Selbst-Verwirklichung. Eine moderne Beschreibung genau dieser ‚Klebrigkeit' des Schattens gibt z. B. Odo Marquard (2000) mit seinem „Satz von der Erhaltung des Negativitätsbedarfs", mit dem er darstellt, dass, selbst bei augenscheinlichen Verbesserungen der tatsächlichen Bedingungen, durch Mechanismen der Aufmerksamkeitslenkung und Bedeutungszuschreibung das Empfinden des Negativen gleich bleibt.

Die Konsequenz der bewussten Anerkennung des Schattens fordert die persönliche Moralität heraus und kann nun aber eben nicht sein, ihn zu bekämpfen und besiegen zu wollen, um ihn endgültig loszuwerden. Vielmehr besteht der ‚Ratschlag' der Analytischen Psychologie in einer bestimmten Form der ‚Integration' des Schattens. Diese wird nicht selten mit der Vokabel des beständigen (inneren) Schattenstreits (Vogel 2015) beschrieben. „Es ist ein eher mit Diplomatie oder Staatskunst zu vergleichendes procedere (...). Vor allem muss man seine (des Schattens, Anm. d. Verf.) Existenz akzeptieren und sie ernstlich berücksichtigen. Zweitens ist erforderlich, sich über seine Eigenschaften und Absichten im Klaren zu sein. Und drittens sind lange und schwierige Verhandlungen unerlässlich" (Jung 1990: 297).

Die Bipolaritäten des Sinns

Schattenpsychologie und Archetypenlehre verweisen auf die Zweiseitigkeit auch des Sinngedankens. Der populär-abendländische Irrtum, die Sinnvokabel vorwiegend bis ausschließlich affirmativ zu konzipieren und nur ins Positive hinein zu deuten und ein oft fast kausal gedachtes bidirektionales Verhältnis zwischen

Sinnerfahrung und Glück/Zufriedenheit zu postulieren, kann vor dem Hintergrund der Konzepte der analytischen Psychologie nicht mehr aufrechterhalten werden. Wir finden Sinndichotomien etwa in der Gegenüberstellung des niemals mit Sinn Versehbaren (Sinnfremden) vs. einer (zumindest potentiellen) Sinnhaftigkeit, in der Möglichkeit eines subjektiven Sinnerlebens vs. kollektiver Sinnzuschreibungen, aber auch, und dies ist im vorliegenden Zusammenhang von besonderer Bedeutung, in moralisch wertvollen vs. anti-moralischen Sinngenerierungen. Wir werden darauf noch zurückkommen. Irvin Yalom (2000) beschreibt folgende Möglichkeiten der Sinnvermittlung:

1. Altruismus (Sinn durch Dienst am Anderen)
2. Hingabe an eine Sache
3. Kreativität (auch in der alltäglichen Arbeit)
4. Hedonismus (Streben nach größtmöglichem Lustgewinn)
5. Selbstverwirklichung

Auch in solchen allgemeinpsychologischen Aufzählungen weisen die einzelnen Sinnkonstruktionen bei genauer Betrachtung helle und dunkle Seiten auf. Psychologische Bipolaritäten zeigen, so Jung, eine Gleichzeitigkeit und psychologische Gleichwertigkeit. Es gilt hier, die Varianten des Dunklen im Sinnkontext aufzuzeigen. So kann etwa eine Sinnkonzeption an sich als „dunkel", also unverständlich, undurchschaubar oder gar unbewusst sein. Der dunkle Sinn ist aber auch der abwesende in Depression und Demoralisierung erlebte Sinn, derjenige Sinn, der gesucht und ersehnt, aber nicht erlebt werden kann, der sich intellektuell und emotional immer wieder entzieht. „Ich habe nichts dagegen, wenn man dies (die „Sinn- und Gegenstandslosigkeit des Lebens", Anm. d. Verf.) als allgemeine Neurose unserer Zeit bezeichnen sollte", meinte Jung dazu (GW 16: § 83.), denn „der Mensch (...) fühlt sich vernichtet, wenn er zusätzlich zu seinem Missgeschick auch noch zugeben muss, dass, was er tut, sinnlos ist" (GW 18/1: § 566).

Die dunkle Seite der Sinnfrage

Belastend und verstörend, ist u.U. zumindest temporär auch die ‚Wirkung' der Sinnfrage schlechthin, ein Faktum, das nicht selten in psychotherapeutischen Kontexten erlebbar ist. Die bewusst gestellte Sinnfrage demontiert evtl. bisherige Illusionen, sie stellt vor die eigene Verantwortlichkeit und führt oft zu einem Aufruf zur Veränderung. Die Sinnfrage hinterfragt die oft selbstverständliche Dauer-Verfügbarkeit des Glücks und konfrontiert mit Begrenztheit und Ohnmacht (vgl. Schnell 2016). Sie ist nicht selten die Grundlage von Empörung und vielleicht auch (positivem oder negativem) Engagement.

Schwierige Behandlungsverläufe bei Patient/-innen mit ‚dunklen' Sinnkonstruktionen zeigen folgende Konstellationen:
- Was subjektiv Sinn vermittelt, ist für sie selbst oder für andere destruktiv.
- Der ein Sinnerleben stiftende persönliche Mythos, das individuelle Lebensskript, kann dunkel sein.
- Sinnerlebnisse sind aktiv-willentlich (etwa durch eine therapeutische Technik) kaum herstellbar, sondern ereignen sich im unbewusst-dunklen Feld von Beziehung.

Schließlich weisen viele tiefenpsychologische Theoriegebäude (wie bekannterweise auch manche spirituelle Traditionen) darauf hin, dass ein bewusstes Erleben von Sinn sich eventuell vorwiegend, vielleicht sogar ausschließlich, in ‚dunklen' Stunden, in Krisenzeiten oder Zeiten des Leides, eröffnen kann: „Wenn alle Stützen und Krücken gebrochen sind und auch nicht die leiseste Rückversicherung irgendwo noch Deckung verspricht, dann erst ist die Möglichkeit gegeben zum Erlebnis eines Archetypus, der sich bisher in der bedeutungsschweren Sinnlosigkeit der Anima verborgen gehalten hatte. Es ist der Archetypus des Sinnes..." (GW 9/1: §66). In der Prozesstheorie der Analytischen Psychologie ist damit, einen alten alchemistischen Terminus aufgreifend, die *nigredo*, die Schwärzung gemeint, die eine tiefe Auseinandersetzung mit dem persönlichen und kollektiven Schatten bedeutet und für das Forstschreiten der Individuation immer wieder vonnöten ist. Diese Sicht erinnert an Schopenhauers Idee des „Sinns im Mangel", denn erst dieser verhelfe uns zur Wahrnehmung. Er stellt dies dar anhand der „... drei größten Güter des Lebens, Gesundheit, Jugend und Freiheit". Erst durch deren Mangel werden sie bewusst. Und er sieht darin die „... gegebene Nachweisung der Negativität aller Befriedigung, also alles Genusses und alles Glückes, im Gegensatz der Positivität des Schmerzes...". So hält Schopenhauer es für richtig, Dunkles, also „Arbeit, Entbehrung, Not und Leiden, gekrönt durch den Tot, als Zweck unseres Lebens zu betrachten" (Schopenhauer 1819: 684). Wie generell kann auch hier eine Beeinflussung Jungs durch die Ideen Schopenhauers durchaus als möglich angenommen werden.

In jüngster Vergangenheit erlebten wir v. a. durch die sog. ‚Corona-Krise' anschaulich diverse Facetten des Dunklen Sinns. Da führt etwa der Kampf gegen das Virus zu unerwarteten Sinnerfahrungen. Nicht nur medizinisches Personal, auch Angestellte von Supermarktketten, LKW-Fahrer/-innen oder Bäckereifachangestellte fühlen ihre Tätigkeit und damit ihre Existenz sinnhaft aufgeladen. Auch das ‚Durchkommen' durch die schweren Zeiten vermittelt Möglichkeiten von Sinnzuschreibungen, und introvertierte Notwendigkeiten wie Rückzug, Stille,

Passivität etc., die in unserer Gesellschaft sonst generell abgewertet werden, werden mit Sinn versehen. ‚Corona' erzwingt eine kompensatorische Bewegung weg vom Aktionismus und der Geschäftigkeit unserer Zeit und wirft den Einzelmenschen auf sich selbst zurück, zwingt zur Selbstreflexion und der potentiell entwicklungsfördernden Frage, was denn nun wirklich wichtig ist. Solche Sinnzuschreibungen sind allerdings nicht unproblematisch, denn, und das ist wichtig zu betonen, sie stellen, unvorsichtig genutzt, eine Verharmlosung oder gar Euphemisierung des (in diesem Fall in einer Pandemie) sich ereignenden menschlichen Leides dar. In unserem Zusammenhang konstelliert sich hier eben eine bestimmte, auch zu anderen Gelegenheiten anzutreffende Art des Dunklen Sinns, nämlich die einer Leidensglorifizierung.

‚Krisengewinnler', seien sie ökonomisch oder narzisstisch motiviert, finden ihren Dunklen Sinn gerade durch das Leid um sie herum. Und natürlich: Die vorübergehende Absurdität des ‚Corona-Alltags' stellt auch die ‚große', die existenzielle Sinnfrage, so wie sie aus Albert Camus' *Die Pest* hinlänglich bekannt ist, ein Buch übrigens, das wie geschaffen ist, als sinnreflektierende Begleitlektüre durch die Corona-Zeiten zu dienen. Die ‚großen Sinnfragen', wenn sie sich in und vielleicht auch nur durch die Konfrontation mit Angst, Leid und Tod ergeben, können eben dadurch ‚Dunkel' genannt werden.

Eine besondere Beachtung gebührt im Zusammenhang mit der dargestellten Bipolarität der Sinnhaftigkeit dem genuin destruktiv-‚bösen' Sinn, dem Un-Sinn in der wörtlichen Bedeutung. Die moderne Sinnforschung, weist darauf hin: „Handlungen werden dann als sinnvoll erfahren, wenn sie übergeordneten Zielen dienen. Zielloses Handeln ist bloße Aktivität..." (Schnell 2016: 27). Dabei scheint es unwesentlich, ob dieses Ziel den geltenden moralischen Vorstellungen entsprechend positiv besetzt ist. Menschen zu töten kann etwa in einem terroristischen Kontext als übergeordneten Zielen dienlich und dadurch sinnbedeutend erlebt werden. Auch die in der modernen Zeit so häufigen Verschwörungserzählungen können als sinnstiftende Schattennarrative verstanden werden. Zu dieser Blickrichtung gehören auch die Forschungen zur sog. „Negativen Kreativität", der „Dark Side of Creativity" (z.B. Cropley u. Cropley 2018, Cropley u.a. 2019). Hier fällt ein weiterer tiefenpsychologischer Mythos: Kreativität und schöpferisches Denken und Handeln entspringen eben nicht per se einer als positiv und gut zu bewertenden Ganzheit, sondern können auch Produkte einseitiger Schattenidentifikationen sein, wie etwa Wissenschaft und Kunst in den Diensten des Nationalsozialismus eindrücklich gezeigt haben. Die Faszination des sog. ‚Dark Tourism' also des Sinnerleben vermittelnden Verbringens der Freizeit an Orten des Grauens und Schreckens (z.B. Stone 2018), weist ebenfalls in diese Richtung. Der Aufruf Ilse Aichingers, „Wir müssen uns selbst misstrauen" (Aichinger 1991), ist hier so zu lesen, dass auch das Sinnerleben von uns nicht als beruhigende Emotion des Guten und Richtigen genommen werden kann.

Schluß

Das alles bedeutet zusammenfassend: Im Sinnerleben liegt bisweilen eine (archetypische) Ergriffenheit. Sinnerleben ist damit ohne moralische Wertigkeit, dem Sinnerleben wird sekundär-kognitiv eine moralische Bedeutung zugeschrieben. Sinnerleben hat einen (sozialen) Ereignischarakter. D.h: Die Bipolarität des Sinns muss ausgehalten werden, nötig ist ein *Schattenstreit* zwischen den Sinnkonstruktionen, ein sich aneinander Reiben der Gegensätze „als möglichem Weg, der nicht Kompromiss sondern Synthese ist" (Vogel 2015: 76) und den Hannah Arendt wohl meint, wenn sie über das „Zusammenleben" mit sich selbst spricht (Arendt 2003). Konsequenz dieses innen-dialogischen Prinzips ist die bewusste Verantwortungsübernahme auch für das, was uns als sinnvoll erscheint.

Literatur

Arendt H (2003) Denktagebuch. München: Piper Verlag.
Aichinger I (1991) Aufruf zum Misstrauen In: Werke in acht Bänden. Frankfurt a. M.: Fischer.
Cropley D, Cropley A (2018) Die Schattenseite der Kreativität. Berlin: Springer.
Cropley DH, Kaufman JC, Cropley AJ (2019) Understanding malevolent creativity. In: Chan J, Thomas K (Hg.): Handbook of Research on Creativity. Cheltenham: Edward Elgar Publishing. 185 – 195.
Jaffé A (1983): Der Mythus vom Sinn im Werk von C.G. Jung. Zürich: Daimon Verlag.
Jung CG (1990) Briefe Bd 1. Olten: Walter Verlag.
Jung CG (1995) Gesammelte Werke. Studienausgabe. Bd 1 – 20. Düsseldorf: Walter Verlag. [GW]
Marquard O (2000) Philosophie des Stattdessen. Reclam.
Neumann E (2009) Mensch und Kultur im Übergang. Düsseldorf: Patmos Verlag.
Riedel I (2009) Die innere Freiheit des Alters. Düsseldorf: Patmos Verlag.
Roesler C (2016) Das Archetypenkonzept C.G. Jungs. Stuttgart: Kohlhammer.
Schnell T (2016): Psychologie des Lebenssinns. Berlin: Springer Verlag.
Schock W (1994) Sinnebenen der Individuation. Zeitschrift für analytische Psychologie 35: 137 – 149.
Schopenhauer A (1819/1993) Die Welt als Wille und Vorstellung II. Zürich: Haffmans.
Stone P (2018) The Darker Side of Travel. The Theory and Practice of Dark Tourism. Bristol: Channel View Publications.
Vogel RT (2015) Das Dunkle im Menschen. Das Schattenkonzept des Analytischen Psychologie.
Vogel RT (2016) Selbst und Tod. In: Frick E, Vogel RT (Hg.): Den Abschied vom Leben verstehen. Stuttgart: Kohlhammer.
Vogel RT (2018) Analytische Psychologie nach C.G. Jung. Stuttgart: Kohlhammer.

v. Franz M-L (2014) Archetypische Dimensionen der Seele. Bd 4. Zürich: Daimon Verlag.
Yalom I (2000) Existenzielle Psychotherapie. Köln: Edition Humanistische Psychologie.

Olivia Mitscherlich

„Unterscheiden“ in Grenzsituationen

Zu Integration, Autonomie und Gedeihen des Selbst in Selbstliebe

'Discerning' in borderline situations

On integration, autonomy, and flourishing of the self in self-love

Zusammenfassung: Welche Rolle spielt Sinn für ein gelingendes Leben von Personen? Diese Frage steht im Hintergrund meiner folgenden Überlegungen. Damit situiere ich mich im weiten Feld der zeitgenössischen Tugendethik: der ethischen Auseinandersetzung mit einer gelingenden Ausübung des personalen Lebens. In meinen Überlegungen maße ich mir keine allgemeingültige Theorie über ein gelingendes – integriertes, autonomes, gedeihendes – Leben von Personen an, um in deren Rahmen die Rolle des Sinns für ein gelingendes Person-Sein zu bestimmen. Ich gehe bescheidener vor und werde ethische Praktiken ins Bewusstsein heben, die uns sozio-kulturell – in biblisch-aufgeklärter Tradition – zur Verfügung stehen: die Selbstliebepraktiken eines ‚Unterscheidens der Geister'. Diese ethischen Praktiken werde ich in zwei Hinsichten befragen: in Bezug auf die besondere Sinnerkenntnis, die sie in Grenzsituationen des Lebens eröffnen (vgl. 2.); und in Bezug auf die metaphysischen Gestalten der Integration, der Autonomie und des Gedeihens, die sie der Selbst-Realisierung vermitteln (vgl. 3.).

Schlüsselwörter: Gelingendes Leben, Selbstliebe, Unterscheiden der Geister, individuell aufgegebenes Selbst-Sein, Selbst-Realisierung, integriertes Selbst, autonomes Selbst, gedeihendes Selbst

Abstract: What role does meaning play for the good life of persons? This question is a background concern for my following considerations. With this, I situate myself within the broad field of contemporary virtue ethics: the ethical engagement with a good exercise of personal life. In my reflections, I do not claim to put forward a general theory of the good – integrated, autonomous, flourishing – personal life in order to determine the role that meaning plays in flourishing as a person. In a more modest approach, I will rather raise awareness of ethical practices that are available to us socio-culturally, in a biblical post-enlightenment tradition – namely: the self-love practices of 'discerning spirits'. These ethical practices will be interrogated in two respects: with regard to the specific in-

https://doi.org/10.1515/9783110787153-010

sight into meaning that they open up in borderline situations of life (cf. 2.); and with regard to the metaphysical forms of integration, autonomy, and flourishing that they afford to self-realization (cf. 3.).

Keywords: Good life, self-love, discernment of spirits, individual destiny, self-realization, integrated self, autonomous self, flourishing self

Einleitung: zu Fragestellung und Methode meiner Überlegungen

Bevor ich mich an die Durchführung dieses Programms mache, möchte ich einen Blick auf den methodischen Ansatz werfen, den ich in die zeitgenössische Tugendethik des gelingenden Lebens einspeise: den Ansatz einer reflektierten Phänomenologie der Selbstliebe. In Gestalt dieses Ansatzes will ich nicht nur eine Alternative zum rationalistischen Paradigma der Tugendethik, sondern auch zu den vorherrschenden Ansätzen innerhalb der nicht-kognitivistischen Tugendethik bahnen: zu den Ansätzen einer pragmatistischen und einer realistischen Gefühlsethik. Indem ich mein methodisches Vorgehen im Folgenden von den genannten Ansätzen abgrenze, sollen zugleich die Gründe dafür verständlich werden, die mich zu der oben skizzierten Eingrenzung meines Themas bewogen haben.

Trotz der Stimmen, die in den letzten Jahren für ein nicht-kognitivistisches Vorgehen eintreten, ist die Tugendethik weiterhin von rationalistischen Ansätzen des gelingenden Lebens dominiert. Die Hauptthese dieser Ansätze bringt Philippa Foot auf den prägnanten Satz, dass, um zu gedeihen, Menschen ebenso auf die Ausbildung von praktischer Vernunft angewiesen seien wie Bienen auf die Ausbildung von Stacheln (vgl. Foot 2004: 66). An dieser These lassen sich die Schwierigkeiten des rationalistischen Vorgehens in der Tugendethik des gelingenden Lebens absehen. Mit dieser Verabsolutierung der praktischen Vernunft zur „Haupttugend" (ebd.: 88) gelingenden Person-Seins spricht Foot dem europäischen Rationalismus das Wort. Diese geschichtliche Verankerung reflektiert Foot jedoch nicht und setzt infolgedessen die Abwertung der leiblichen und emotionalen Aspekte unseres Person-Seins fort, die diese Tradition bestimmt (vgl. Gamm 2009).

Gegenüber dieser rationalistischen Engführung rücken nicht-kognitivistische Ansätze der Tugendethik in den letzten Jahren die emotionalen und sympathetischen Quellen der praktischen Vernunft in den Blick (vgl. exemplarisch Engelen 2003; Frankfurt 2005: 61 f.). Wenn ich mir im Folgenden meinerseits den Ansatz einer reflektierten Phänomenologie der Selbstliebe zur Aufgabe mache, dann ist es mir nicht darum zu tun, im Sinne dieses non-kognitivistischen Vorgehens den Wechsel von der praktischen Vernunft zur Selbstliebe als der ‚Kardinaltugend' vorzunehmen, die das individuelle Person-Sein gedeihen lasse. Beide prominenten Ansätze der Gefühlsethik, die für das Lieben als ‚Haupttugend' eintreten, nehmen in ihren Vorstellungen eines gedeihenden Person-Seins nämlich – wie Foot – die Grenzen nicht ernst genug, die ihrem philosophischen Wissen durch ihre eigene Zeitlichkeit gesetzt sind. Auf Seiten einer realistischen Gefühlsethik geht Christine Tappolet in Anschluss an Max Scheler davon aus, dass Wertverhalte metaphysische Eigenschaften von Situationen sind und dass die Emotionen die Erkenntnisformen darstellen, die – und nur die – ebendiese Eigenschaften zugänglich machen (vgl. Tappolet 2009). Scheler selbst entwirft eine Theorie des menschlichen Gedeihens auf der Grundlage seiner realistischen Theorie des Wertfühlens. Um zu gedeihen, sind Menschen nach Scheler auf die Ausbildung einer „objektiv rechte[n] Ordnung" ihres Liebens und Hassens angewiesen (Scheler 2000: 347). Die Grenzen dieses Ansatzes bestehen in der Voraussetzung, dass es in einer Situation nur eine korrekte Emotion geben könne (vgl. Döring 2009: 48 f.). Abgeblendet sind darin die sozio-kulturellen Praktiken, die eine Situation und das emotionale Erleben in der Situation mitbestimmen. Infolgedessen laufen Vertreter/-innen der realistischen Gefühlsethik Gefahr, das eigene Fühlen zum richtigen Fühlen zu verabsolutieren.

Im Unterschied zur realistischen Gefühlsethik reflektieren Vertreter/-innen einer pragmatistischen Gefühlsethik die Vermittlung des emotionalen und erotischen Erlebens durch sozio-kulturell hervorgebrachte Liebespraktiken: des Sich-Sorgens (vgl. Frankfurt 2005) oder des Teilens eines Lebens (vgl. Krebs 2015: 226–229). Den pragmatistischen Gedanken von der Konstitution des erotischen Erlebens durch die Liebespraktiken des Sich-Sorgens spitzt Harry Frankfurt auf die These zu, dass wir „die Dinge nicht zwangsläufig deshalb [lieben; OMS], *weil* wir ihren Wert erkennen", sondern dass vielmehr „das, was wir lieben, notwendig an Wert für uns [*gewinnt*], *weil* wir es lieben" (Frankfurt 2005: 43). Vor dem Hintergrund dieser pragmatistischen Liebestheorie tritt Frankfurt für ein formales Verständnis menschlichen Gedeihens ein: dass Menschen gedeihen, wenn sie das, was sie – ohne Wissen von dessen inhärenten Wert – lieben, „entschlossen" lieben (ebd.: 103). Mit der Theorie von der sozio-kulturellen Konstruktion des emotionalen und erotischen Erlebens ist die pragmatistische Emotions- und Liebesethik der metaphysischen Voranname verpflichtet, dass – in den Worten von Angelika Krebs – „*alles* Geistige und Seelische in unserem Leben auf Handlungen und ihre Normierungen zurück[geht]" (Krebs 2015: 215; Herv. OMS). Mit dieser Voraussetzung verstrickt sich die pragmatistische Emotions- und Liebesethik jedoch nicht nur in Selbstwidersprüche, da sie ihre eigene Zeitlichkeit auf methodologischer Ebene nicht ernst genug nimmt: wenn alles Erkennen durch sozio-kulturelle Handlungen vermittelt wäre, dann ließe sich nämlich gerade keine universalgültige Meta-Theorie über alles Erkennen aufstellen. Sie greift darüber hinaus auch beim Verständnis des erotischen Erlebens und des menschlichen Gedeihens zu kurz. Wer wie Frankfurt das erotische Erleben auf Liebespraktiken zurückführt, wird dem subjektiven Erleben Liebender nicht gerecht: in den Liebespraktiken nicht nur Bedeutungszusammenhänge zu konstruieren, sondern in deren Rahmen vielmehr auch Sinn zu erfahren, den inneren Wert des Geliebten zu erkennen. Und wer wie Frankfurt menschliches Gedeihen in der Entschlossenheit wertblinder Liebespraktiken findet, der blendet die Gefahren ab, die für das menschliche Gedeihen gerade von wertblinder Entschlossenheit ausgehen können: etwa im entschlossenen Festhalten an lang eingeübten Ressentiments zu übersehen, worum es individuell hier und jetzt eigentlich geht (vgl. ausführlicher Abschnitt 2). Angesichts dieser Schwierigkeiten ist gegenüber der pragmatistischen Liebesethik darauf zu bestehen, dass uns inmitten der Zeit ein Erkenntnisstandpunkt auch noch für eine formale Theorie über das Gedeihen aller Menschen entzogen ist.

Meinerseits möchte ich ethisches Wissen über gedeihendes Person-Sein in den methodologischen Grenzen erreichen, die mir durch meine eigene Geschichtlichkeit gezogen sind. Zu diesem Zweck bahne ich in Gestalt meines Ansatzes einer reflektierten Phänomenologie einen dritten Weg innerhalb der nichtkognitivistischen Sterbensethik. Inhaltlich mache ich mir besondere sozio-kulturell tradierte Selbstsorgepraktiken zum Gegenstand: die Urteilspraktiken eines ‚Unterscheidens der Geister', in denen wir Selbstliebe ausüben können. In methodischer Hinsicht übernehme ich bewusst meine geschichtliche Bindung an die Selbstliebepraktiken des ‚Unterscheidens', um letztere ‚von innen' auszuleuchten. So reflektiere ich zunächst – mit der pragmatistischen gegen die realistische Gefühlsethik – die Vermittlung des emotionalen und erotischen Erlebens durch sozio-kulturelle Praktiken. In der weiteren, methodologischen Ausgestaltung meiner Liebesethik widersetze ich mich jedoch der pragmatistischen Überhöhung der sozio-kulturellen Vermittlung zur Konstruktion des emotionalen Erlebens. Im Wissen um die Grenzen, die dem philosophischen Erkennen unter den Bedingungen der Zeit gesetzt sind, halte ich vielmehr die metaphysische Frage nach dem Primat von Erkenntnissubjekt oder -objekt offen. Damit enthalte ich mich in meinem methodischen Vorgehen metaphysischer Vorannahmen über die Realität bzw. die pragmatische Konstruktion der begegnenden Wertverhalte – die in die oben skizzierten Schwierigkeiten führen. Methodisch kann ich die Primatfragen offenhalten, indem ich – im Sinne des „höchsten Grundsatzes der Phänomenologie" – die Korrelation bzw. den „Zusammenhang zwischen dem Wesen des Gegenstands und dem Wesen des intentionalen Erlebnisses" (Scheler 1927: 272) ins Auge fasse. Im Wissen um die geschichtliche Vermittlung des subjektiven

Erlebens heißt das genauer: nach dem Zueinander zwischen dem – durch die sozio-kulturellen Praktiken des ‚Unterscheidens‘ vermittelten – subjektiven Erlebens der Selbstliebe und der Art des In-Erscheinung-Tretens des Begegnenden zu fragen (An diesem Punkt gehe ich auch über Hans Joas „affirmative Genealogie“ hinaus, die dem pragmatistischen Modell der sozio-kulturellen Konstruktion von Bedeutungen verpflichtet bleibt (vgl. Joas 2015: 147–203).

Auf diese Weise wird es mir möglich, das ‚Unterscheiden‘ als eine besondere sozio-kulturelle Urteilspraxis aufzuzeigen, in der nicht nur Selbstliebe gelebt werden kann, sondern die mit der Selbstliebe zu spezifischen Erfahrungen des Begegnenden befähigt: zu den Sinnerfahrungen des Herausgefordert-Werdens durch konkrete ‚Gebote der Stunde‘, die in Selbstliebe gemacht werden können. Vor dem Hintergrund dieser Sinnkorrelation kann ich zeigen, dass die spezifischen Formen der Integration, der Autonomie und des Gedeihens, die in den Selbstliebepraktiken des ‚Unterscheidens‘ gelebt werden, nicht nur funktionaler, sondern metaphysischer Natur sind: vermittelt durch das individuell aufgegebene Selbst-Sein.

In normativer Hinsicht geht es mir mit dem Ansatz einer reflektierten Phänomenologie darum, durch theoretisches Verstehen Verantwortung für das Fortbestehen des ‚Unterscheidens‘ zu übernehmen. Indem wir zur Selbstliebe nämlich durch die sozio-kulturellen Praktiken des ‚Unterscheidens‘ befähigt werden, steht uns diese existenzielle Grundhaltung mitsamt ihrer genuinen Potenziale der Selbst-Werdung – zumindest in der Gestalt, die ich ins Bewusstsein hebe – nur solange offen, wie wir ebendiese Praktiken bewahren und kultivieren.

Der Sinnbezug der Selbstliebepraktiken des ‚Unterscheidens‘ in Grenzsituationen des Lebens

Im ersten Schritt meiner Überlegungen möchte ich dafür eintreten, dass in Grenzsituationen des Lebens in Gestalt der Urteilspraktiken eines ‚Unterscheidens der Geister‘ ein *ethos* der Selbstliebe ausgeübt wird und dass die im Modus des ‚Unterscheidens‘ praktizierte Selbstliebe zu einer spezifischen Sinnkorrelation befähigt: zum In-die-Pflicht-Genommen-Werden durch konkrete ‚Forderungen der Stunde‘.

Philosophisch verfügen wir inmitten des Lebens zwar über keinen Standpunkt, um das menschliche Leben als Ganzes zu überblicken – und Wissen über dessen Gedeihen zu generieren. Wohl jedoch ist es inmitten des Lebens möglich, Scharnierstellen der individuellen Lebensgestaltung auszumachen. Diese Scharnierstellen finde ich in Anschluss an Karl Jaspers in praktisch-existenziellen

Grenzsituationen des Lebens (vgl. Jaspers 1932/1994: 201–209). Zu denken wäre etwa an Situationen, die von schwerer Erkrankung, dem Bevorstehen des Todes, eigener Schuld oder auch von Begegnungen der Liebe bestimmt sind. Solche praktisch-existenziellen Grenzsituationen zeichnen sich – in den Worten von Theda Rehbock – durch ein „Durchbrechen der gewohnheitsmäßigen Normalität des Lebens“ (Rehbock 2005: 37) aus. Sie sind „nicht überschaubar“ wie Jaspers selbst schreibt (Jaspers 1932/1994: 203). Allgemeinbegriffe – wie Leben, Gesundheit, Gedeihen – greifen bei ihrer Bestimmung zu kurz; ‚Leitbilder‘ (Zum Begriff des ‚Leitbildes‘ in der Medizinethik vgl. Kersting 2017). einer guten Lebensführung treten in Grenzsituationen in ihrer Fraglichkeit und Rückhaltlosigkeit hervor. Indem eingeübte Muster des Lebens und Erlebens ihre bisherige Selbstverständlichkeit verlieren, begegnen in Grenzsituationen unterschiedlichste, oft untereinander kollidierende Anforderungen an unsere individuelle Lebensgestaltung. So können sich etwa Gebärende – wenn sich die Geburt durch Komplikationen plötzlich zu einer Grenzsituation steigert – als von den kollidierenden Forderungen in die Pflicht genommen erfahren, mit ihrem lang gehegten ‚Leitbild‘ einer ‚natürlichen Geburt‘ zu brechen und sich einem Kaiserschnitt zu unterziehen; und sich im Gespür für unsere eigene Leiblichkeit dem ärztlichen Rat gerade zu widersetzen. Angesichts des Infragestehens bisheriger Lebensmuster gewinnt das Verhalten zu den Lebensanforderungen, die in Grenzsituationen auftreten, einen doppelten Status: im Umgang mit ebendiesen Anforderungen wird zusammen mit der konkreten Lebenssituation auch über die Gestalt des künftigen Lebens entschieden.

Im Unterschied zu Jaspers selbst setze ich an den Grenzsituationen des Lebens nicht an, um existenzielles Wissen über eine Lebensform ins Bewusstsein zu heben, die das Mensch-Sein von seinen Grenzsituationen her gedeihen lässt (vgl. Jaspers 1932/1994: 204–209). In seiner Tugendethik eines Werdens zur Existenz nimmt Jaspers die meta-philosophischen Konsequenzen seiner eigenen Einsicht in das Phänomen der Grenzsituation nämlich nicht ernst genug: dass die philosophische Ethik mit den Grenzsituationen Situationen des Mensch-Seins begegnet, die sich jedweder Bestimmung durch Allgemeinbegriffe und damit zugleich jedem ‚Leitbild‘ der – guten, gelingenden, gedeihenden – Lebensführung widersetzen. Mir ist es vielmehr darum zu tun, eine sozio-kulturell tradierte Urteilspraxis ins Bewusstsein zu heben, die wir in Grenzsituationen nicht – um willen der natürlichen Bestimmung unseres Mensch-Seins – ausüben *müssen*, sondern vielmehr ausüben *können:* die auf den ersten Blick unscheinbare Urteilspraxis, inmitten der Grenzsituationen zusammen mit Freund/-innen die Anforderungen zu reflektieren und zu kritisieren, die in ihnen an uns ergehen (Zur dialogischen Anlage des ‚Unterscheidens‘ vgl. ausführlicher Mitscherlich-Schönherr 2019: 109 f.). Diese reflektierende Urteilspraxis möchte ich im Rückgriff auf einen Paulinischen Begriff als ‚Unterscheiden der Geister‘ (vgl. 1 Kor 12,10) bezeichnen. Das reflektierende Urteilen des ‚Unterscheidens‘ zeichnet sich durch seine Rückhaltlosigkeit aus. Es unterscheidet sich darin von Formen eines bestimmenden Urteilens durch Subsumtion unter Allgemeinbegriffe (zum reflektierenden und bestimmenden Urteilen vgl. Kant 1793/1983: B XXVI). Im ‚Unterscheiden‘ werden keine ‚Leitbilder‘ eines guten, gelingenden oder gedeihenden Lebens in Anspruch genommen, um die begegnenden Lebensforderungen in Bezug auf ihre Gutheit zu bestimmen. Das ‚Unterscheiden‘ setzt überhaupt nicht an den Inhalten dieser Forderungen, sondern vielmehr an der *emotionalen Verfasstheit* unseres Gefordert-Werdens an. Ohne ‚Leitbild‘ ist es gleichwohl nicht willkürlich. Das ‚Unterscheiden‘ bildet vielmehr eine Praxis, ein erotisches In-die-Pflicht-Genommen-Werden von emotionalen Verstrickungen zu scheiden. Als parteiliche Praxis, in der das eigene Lieben bejaht bzw. geliebt wird, formt es – mit Harry Frankfurt gesprochen – eine Praxis der Selbstliebe (vgl. Frankfurt 2005: 92). Zurückgewiesen wird ein narzisstisches Getrieben-Werden durch diffuse Gefühlszustände der Angst, durch Ressentiments sowie durch Werturteile und ‚Leitbilder‘ des Guten, die in der Vergangenheit ausgebildet worden sind. Damit wird in der Grenzsituation das Etablieren von solchen Lebensmustern unterlaufen, die in die Wiederholung des immer gleichen Fühlens und Handelns zwingen; und uns zugleich übersehen lassen, worum es für uns im hier und jetzt unseres Lebens eigentlich ginge. Bejaht wird dagegen das In-die-Pflicht-Genommen-Werden durch das eigene Lieben in der konkreten Situation, in der man sich hier und jetzt befindet.

Um die spezifische Sinnkorrelation und die genuinen Lebensmuster zu verstehen, die im ‚unterscheidenden‘ Bejahen des eigenen Liebens etabliert werden, ist von ebendiesem Lieben erster Ordnung auszugehen. Unter dem Lieben erster Ordnung – das im ‚Unterscheiden‘ bejahend übernommen wird – verstehe ich Liebesereignisse: die Ereignisse des emotionalen Affiziert-Werdens durch begegnende Wertverhalte, die durch subjektive Akte des erotischen Sich-Öffnens ermöglicht werden. In Bezug auf das emotionale Affiziert-Werden durch begegnende Wertverhalte denke ich an die Fälle, die die realistische Gefühlsethik vor Augen hat: das Fühlen der Gerechtigkeit einer Handlung, der Grazie einer Bewegung oder der Schönheit eines Morgens. Im Unterschied zur realistischen Gefühlsethik – in der oben erwähnten Fassung von Tappolet – gehe ich davon aus, dass die Angemessenheit der Emotionen nicht von den begegnenden Wertqualitäten, sondern durch subjektive Akte des Liebens gestiftet wird. Indem wir uns erotisch öffnen, ist unser Fühlen gut verfasst und unsere Emotionen dem Begegnenden angemessen. Ereignisse der Liebe stellen sich damit als besondere Begegnungsereignisse dar. Eine Person, die sich in einer konkreten Lebenssituation erotisch öffnet, sieht sich weder mit unzusammenhängenden, wertneutralen Daten konfrontiert noch in ihrem emotionalen Erleben durch Bedeutungszusammenhängen aus ihrer Vergangenheit bedingt, sondern wird emotional von den Wertverhalten ebendieser Situation affiziert (Wenn John L. Mackie Werte als absonderliche Entitäten ohne Bezug zu allem übrigen im Universum bezeichnet, dann verabsolutiert er unter der Hand das naturwissenschaftliche Weltbild; vgl. Mackie 1986: insb. Teil I). Robert Spaemann schreibt über derartige Begegnungen der Liebe, dass in ihnen „das Wirkliche" für die liebende Person „wirklich wird" (Spaemann 1989: 124 f.). Als Beispiele wäre etwa an ein Ereignis der Naturliebe zu denken, in dem eine Naturliebhaberin von der Erhabenheit eines Gebirgszuges angesprochen wird; oder an eine Begegnung in Freundschaft, in der Freund/-innen emotional das in sich wertvolle Dasein des Anderen erfassen.

Indem nun im ‚Unterscheiden' das eigene Lieben erster Ordnung bejaht wird, wird ein erotisches Sich-Öffnen auf der Ebene der individuellen Existenz ausgeübt: ein existenzielles Sich-Öffnen für das eigene Lieben. Damit stiftet der Vollzug des ‚Unterscheidens' eine Korrelation zwischen der individuellen Existenz und den Sinnqualitäten, die diese Situation birgt. Indem wir uns ‚unterscheidend' in einer Grenzsituation des Lebens für unser eigenes Lieben öffnen, werden wir nämlich emotional durch die konkreten ‚Forderungen der Stunde' affizierbar, die von den Wertverhalten ebendieser Lebenssituation ausgehen. In ein Leben, in dem die Forderungen unterschieden werden, die sich in seinen Grenzsituationen zu Wort melden, bricht damit Sinn in Gestalt der ‚Gebote' bzw. der „demands of the situation" (Frankl 1972/2016: 24) ein, die von den Wertqualitäten ebendieser Situationen an uns ergehen. Indem die konkreten ‚Forderungen der Stunde' verstanden und als orientierende Maßstäbe der Lebensführung bejaht werden, wird im ‚Unterscheiden' inmitten der Grenzsituation des Lebens eine spezifische Lebensform ausgebildet. Verstrickungen in überkommene Muster der Lebensführung werden unterlaufen und die individuelle Lebensgestaltungen wird am Widerfahrenden ausgerichtet: an dem besonderen Mensch-Sein, das uns in Grenzsituationen, in denen wir uns selbst lieben, in Gestalt der konkreten ‚Forderungen der Stunde' aufgegeben ist – ohne dass wir diskursives Wissen davon hätten.

Im Unterschied zu Frankl möchte ich auch das *ethos*, in der Lebensführung an den ‚Geboten der Stunde' Maß zu nehmen, nicht zur Quelle menschlichen Gedeihens erklären (vgl. ebd.: 17). Mit dieser These blendet Frankl seine eigene geschichtliche Bindung an ebendieses *ethos* ab – und läuft in der Überdehnung seines Wissensanspruchs Gefahr, von einer Praxis der Selbstliebe in eine Praxis der ‚Eigenliebe' zu verkehren: in eine Praxis, das eigene Leben im Ausgang von dem ‚Leitbild' zu führen, das irgendwann in der Vergangenheit aufgestellt wurde – und das nun ‚Selbsttranszendenz zum Sinn' heißt. Auch dieses ‚Leitbild' kann aber in einer konkreten Grenzsituation den Blick dafür verstellen, worum es hier und jetzt eigentlich geht: etwa nicht in Gelassenheit, sondern in Aufruhr gegen die Sinnlosigkeit eines Todes zu sterben, der viel zu früh für einen kommt. Im Wissen um meine eigene Geschichtlichkeit halte ich im Folgenden die Frage nach dem guten Mensch-Sein offen und frage – wie einleitend angekündigt – nicht nach der Funktion des ‚Unterscheidens‘ für menschliches Gedeihen, sondern befrage diese Selbstliebepraxis vielmehr von ‚innen heraus‘ nach der genuinen Gestalt des Selbst-Seins, das sich in ihrem Vollzug konstituiert.

Integration, Autonomie und Gedeihen des Selbst im Modus des ‚Unterscheidens‘

Bevor ich mich mit den Formen der Integration, der Autonomie und des Gedeihens auseinandersetzen kann, die das ‚Unterscheiden‘ dem individuellen Selbst-Sein eröffnet, muss ich zunächst auf das Selbst-Verhältnis blicken, das diese Selbstliebepraxis bestimmt.

Das Selbst-Verhältnis der Selbstliebepraktiken des ‚Unterscheidens‘

Das ‚Unterscheiden‘ steht in einem doppelten Verhältnis zum Selbst derjenigen, die es ausüben. Zum einen wird im ‚Unterscheiden‘ ein spezifisches Verständnis des eigenen Selbst vorausgesetzt: ein anthropologisches Verständnis des eigenen Selbst-Seins, unter dessen Bedingung diese rückhaltlose Lebensführung allererst möglich wird. Zum anderen wird im Vollzug des ‚Unterscheidens‘ das reale Selbst-Sein seiner Subjekte mit hervorgebracht.

In der rückhaltlosen Lebensführung des ‚Unterscheidens‘ wird das eigene Selbst implizit oder explizit als ‚unergründlich‘ – im Sinne von Helmuth Plessner – angesprochen (vgl. Plessner 1931/1981: 175–185). Dabei meint, das eigene Selbst als ‚unergründlich‘ anzusprechen, nicht, Denkverbote zu errichten und jegliche Bestimmung zurückzuweisen – wodurch gar nichts gesagt wäre. Es meint vielmehr, in allen Versuchen, Wissen vom eigenen Selbst zu erreichen, dessen Wesen oder Substanz gegenüber Allgemeinbestimmungen offenzuhalten. Wenn eine ‚unterscheidende‘ Person ihr eigenes Selbst als ‚unergründlich‘ adressiert, dann fasst sie mit anderen Worten zunächst den Umstand ins Auge, dass sie sich nicht vollständig durchsichtig ist.

Eine ‚unterscheidende' Person hält die Substanz des eigenen Selbst in der Frage, indem sie ein integratives, geschichtliches Verständnis des eigenen Selbst vertritt. Integrativ ist ihr Selbst-Verständnis, indem es – im Sinne von Helmuth Plessners Philosophischer Anthropologie – heterogene Aspekte des personalen Lebens verschränkt, anstatt einzelne Aspekte zu verabsolutieren (vgl. Plessner 1928/1975: insb. 288–293). In das Verständnis des eigenen Selbst werden bewusst zugängliche und vor-bewusste, ideale und reale, individuelle und mit Anderen geteilte Aspekte des personalen Lebens integriert (vgl. Brüntrup 2014). Es werden unmittelbare, erstpersonale Selbst-Erfahrungen – der leiblichen Gesamtverfassung, des seelischen Gestimmtseins und des emotionalen Affiziert-Werdens – genauso berücksichtigt wie drittpersonal zugängliche, körperliche Dispositionen und Charakteranlagen (vgl. Ricœur 2005: 150 und 390 f.). Zugleich wird das eigene Selbst-Sein nicht auf das Dasein in den Grenzen des eigenen Körperleibs reduziert, sondern darin auch das Leben mit den Anderen einbezogen: geteilte, dialogische Praktiken und sozio-kulturell tradierte Bedeutungszusammenhänge (vgl. ebd.: 396). Geschichtlich ist das Verständnis ihres „realen Selbst" (vgl. Brüntrup 2014), das ‚unterscheidende' Personen in Anspruch nehmen. Indem sie die Substanz ihres Selbst in der Frage halten, stellt sich ihnen die Einheit der heterogenen Aspekte ihres Selbst-Seins als geschichtlich konstituierte Einheit dar. Im Lichte ihrer unergründlichen Substanz sprechen sie ihr ‚reales Selbst' als die besondere Gestalt an, die sie in den konkreten Lebenssituationen im Umgang mit den an sie ergehenden Lebensanforderungen ausbilden.

Mit der Auffassung ihres eigenen Selbst als ‚unergründlich' adressieren ‚unterscheidende' Personen die anthropologischen Voraussetzungen ihrer Selbstliebepraktiken. Sie reflektieren darin den Umstand, dass sie durch keine vorgegebenen Lebensmuster – der menschlichen Gattung oder ihres Kulturkreises – determiniert, sondern in der Offenheit ihres Wesens zu individueller Selbst-Werdung freigesetzt sind. Mit dieser Befähigung zum individuellen Selbst-Werden fassen sie die anthropologische Bedingung ins Auge, unter der es ihnen möglich ist, im Rückgriff auf die sozio-kulturellen Urteilspraktiken des ‚Unterscheidens' von den konkreten ‚Geboten der Stunde' her zu leben. Indem sie ihr eigenes Selbst in der Frage halten, enthalten sie sich zugleich des naturalistischen Fehlschlusses, aus der ‚Unergründlichkeit' des menschlichen Selbst die Allgemeingültigkeit ihrer eigenen, ethischen Lebenspraxis ableiten zu wollen. Sie wissen, dass die Rückhaltlosigkeit unseres Selbst-Seins uns freisetzt, aber nicht zwingt, unsere Lebensführung ‚unterscheidend' an den ‚Geboten der Stunde' auszurichten.

Im Vollzug des ‚Unterscheidens' wird das eigene Selbst nicht nur in seinem ‚unergründlichen' Wesen adressiert, sondern zugleich auch in seiner geschichtlichen Gestalt mit-konstituiert. Genauer werden im ‚Unterscheiden' die idealen Aspekte des realen Selbst auf eine genuin erotische Weise realisiert. Das ‚Unterscheiden‘ der Lebensanforderungen, die in einer konkreten Situation an uns ergehen, ist für die geschichtliche Selbst-Werdung von Belang, da darin konkrete Lebensmöglichkeiten ergriffen bzw. ausgeschieden werden. Zusammen mit den Lebensanforderungen werden die Selbst-Ideale ‚unterschieden‘, die diese Lebensoptionen bestimmen. Indem das In-die-Pflicht-Genommen-Werden durch Ängste, Ressentiments und Werturteile zurückgewiesen wird, werden die darin präsenten Selbst-Bilder als verfehlt abgelehnt. Und indem die ‚Gebote der Stunde‘ gehört und übernommen werden, wird das ideale Selbst, in das diese Forderungen hineinrufen, als das eigene, wahre Selbst bejaht (vgl. Scheler 2000: 353). Damit wird das in den ‚Forderungen der Stunde‘ aufgegebene, ideale Selbst als das Gesetz übernommen, das die eigene Selbst-Realisierung anleitet – ohne dass die ‚unterscheidende‘ Person diskursives Wissen von ihrem wahren Selbst beanspruchte.

Integration, Autonomie und Gedeihen des im Modus des ‚Unterscheidens‘ realisierten Selbst

Im letzten Abschnitt meiner Überlegungen kann ich nun nach den Gestalten der Integration, der Autonomie und des Gedeihens fragen, die das reale Selbst im Modus des ‚Unterscheidens‘ gewinnt. Ich möchte dafür eintreten, dass das ‚Unterscheiden‘ dem realen Selbst keine bloß funktionalen, sondern vielmehr metaphysisch bestimmte Formen der Integration, Autonomie und Gedeihen eröffnet – ohne dass es dabei auf eine positive Bestimmung eigenen Selbst zurückgriffe, das sich inmitten der Zeit unserem Erkennen entzieht.

Um die genuinen Formen der Integration zu verstehen, die das reale Selbst im ‚Unterscheiden‘ gewinnt, möchte ich nochmals auf die Konstitution von dessen idealen Aspekten im Vollzug dieser Selbstliebepraktiken blicken. In meinen bisherigen Überlegungen habe ich das Verhältnis von realem Selbst und Wirklichkeit noch abgeblendet, das im ‚Unterscheiden‘ ausgebildet wird. Im Rückgriff auf einen Begriff von Ernst Tugendhat lässt sich dieses Wirklichkeitsverhältnis als ein Verhältnis der „Entzentrierung“ (Tugendhat 1998/2001: 88) verstehen. Das in der konkreten Lebenssituation Gebotene wird als die Gestalt des Mensch-Seins übernommen, die individuell im Ganzen der Wirklichkeit aufgegeben ist. Von den begegnenden ‚Geboten der Stunde‘ her erfährt das reale Selbst seine metaphysische Integration: es wird in umfassende Sinnzusammenhänge eingerückt – von denen wir inmitten des Lebens freilich wiederum kein theoretisches Wissen haben. Zusammen mit dieser metaphysischen Integration erfährt das reale Selbst im Modus des ‚Unterscheidens‘ auch seine funktionale Integration. Darunter verstehe ich die interne Integration von unterschiedlichen Aspekten des eigenen Person-Seins in das reale Selbst. In negativer Hinsicht werden zusammen mit überkommenen Ängsten, Ressentiments und ‚Leitbildern' Verhärtungen in der Lebensführung überwunden: theoretische und praktische Festlegungen auf einseitige Vorstellungen vom eigenen Selbst-Sein, die desintegrierend wirken können, indem sie Aspekte des eigenen Selbst-Seins unterdrücken. In positiver Hinsicht wird die Selbst-Realisierung mit der Orientierung an den ‚Forderungen der Stunde' am individuell aufgegebenen Selbst ausgerichtet und damit nicht willkürlich, sondern im Lichte eines Gesetzes ausgeübt – das in der Situation freilich nicht gewusst, sondern allererst gesucht wird.

Im Modus des ‚Unterscheidens' wird der Selbst-Konstitution darüber hinaus eine genuine Form der Autonomie erschlossen. Dabei handelt es sich freilich nicht um die Autonomie einer Lebensführung nach Plan – in der etwa John Rawls die Quelle eines gelingenden Lebens findet (vgl. Rawls 1971: 445 ff.). Solch eine Vorstellung des autonomen Selbst hätte allein schon die fremden Kontrahenten der Lebensplanung innerhalb des eigenen Selbst gegen sich: die vor-bewussten, körper-leiblichen Aspekte genauso wie die sozio-kulturell vorgegebenen Aspekte der eigenen Selbst-Werdung. Autonomie wird vielmehr in der Rückhaltlosigkeit der Selbstliebe-Praxis des ‚Unterscheidens' erreicht. Im ‚Unterscheiden' ist das ‚unterscheidende' Selbst autonom, indem es im Bewusstsein seiner eigenen Fraglichkeit das eigene Lieben aus freien Stücken bejaht. Es ist autonom, indem es die eigene Lebensführung in freier Hingabe an den ‚Geboten der Stunde' ausrichtet, die sich ihm im Lieben zeigen.

Und schließlich eröffnet das ‚Unterscheiden' dem Selbst auch spezifische Formen des Gedeihens. Dabei reduziert sich das Gedeihen, das das ‚Unterscheiden' vermittelt, nicht auf ein funktionales Gedeihen, sondern umfasst wiederum auch metaphysische Aspekte. Unter dem metaphysischen Gedeihen des realen Selbst verstehe ich sein Gedeihen im Sinne seiner Bestimmung: als ein Werden zu sich selbst. Dabei bemisst sich das metaphysische Gedeihen freilich an keiner hypostasierten, natürlichen Bestimmung unseres Mensch-Seins, sondern vielmehr an der „individuellen Bestimmung" (Scheler 2000: 353) des in der Situation individuell aufgegebenen Selbst-Seins. Im Modus des ‚Unterscheidens' gedeiht das reale Selbst mit anderen Worten in metaphysischer Hinsicht nach Maßgabe des besonderen Selbst-Seins, das ihm in den ‚Forderungen der Stunde' abverlangt ist, das es als sein ‚wahres Selbst' bejaht und als Gesetz seiner Lebensführung übernimmt. Dabei ist dieses metaphysische Werden zu sich selbst von keinem nüchternen Erkenntnisstandpunkt, sondern allein von dem Erkenntnisstandpunkt der Liebe zugänglich – der im Vollzug des ‚Unterscheidens' eingenommen wird. Das Verstehen und Bejahen des individuell aufgegebenen Selbst-Seins und Gedeihen als reales Selbst im Sinne dieser individuellen Bestimmung greifen folglich ineinander. Zusammen mit diesem metaphysischen Gedeihen eröffnet das ‚Unterscheiden‘ dem realen Selbst wiederum funktionale Formen des Gedeihens. In funktionaler Hinsicht gedeiht es, indem es – mit Harry Frankfurt gesprochen – innere Kohärenz und Entschlossenheit gewinnt (vgl. Frankfurt 2005: 103–105). Im Modus des ‚Unterscheidens‘ werden die Konflikte zwischen unterschiedlichen Lebensanforderungen in Grenzsituationen des Lebens aufgelöst und die ‚Gebote der Stunde‘ entschlossen übernommen.

Literatur

Brüntrup G (2014) Reales und ideales Selbst. In: Viertbauer K, Kögerler R (Hg.) Das autonome Subjekt. Eine Denkform in Bedrängnis. Regensburg: Friedrich Pustet. 135–158.

Döring SA (2009) Allgemeine Einleitung: Philosophie der Gefühle heute. In: Dies. (Hg.) Philosophie der Gefühle. Frankfurt a. M.: Suhrkamp. 12–68.

Engelen EM (2003) Erkenntnis und Liebe. Zur fundierenden Rolle des Gefühls bei den Leistungen der Vernunft. Göttingen: Vandenhoeck & Ruprecht.

Foot P (2004) Die Natur des Guten. Frankfurt a. M.: Suhrkamp.

Frankfurt H (2005) Gründe der Liebe. Frankfurt a. M.: Suhrkamp.

Frankl V (1972/2016) Der Wille zum Sinn. Bern: Hogrefe.

Gamm G (2009) Am Leitfaden des Leibes. In: Ders. Philosophie im Zeitalter der Extreme. Eine Geschichte der Philosophie im 20. Jahrhundert. Darmstadt: Wiss. Buchges. 60–72.

Jaspers K (1932/1994) Philosophie. Bd. II: Existenzerhellung. München: Piper.

Joas H (2015) Die Sakralität der Person. Eine neue Genealogie der Menschenrechte. Berlin: Suhrkamp.

Kant I (1793/1983) Kritik der Urteilskraft. In: Weischedel W (Hg.) Imannuel Kant Werke. Bd. 8. Darmstadt: Wiss. Buchges. 233–620.

Krebs A (2015) Zwischen Ich und Du. Eine dialogische Philosophie der Liebe. Berlin: Suhrkamp.

Mackie JL (1986) Ethik. Die Erfindung des moralisch Richtigen und Falschen. Stuttgart: Reclam.

Mitscherlich-Schönherr O (2019) Das Lieben im Sterben. Eine verstehende Liebesethik des Sterbens in Selbstliebe. In: Dies. (Hg.) Gelingendes Sterben. Zeitgenössische Theorien im interdisziplinären Dialog. Berlin: de Gruyter. 101–128.

Plessner H (1928/1975) Die Stufen des Organischen und der Mensch. Berlin/New York: de Gruyter.

Plessner H (1931/1981) Macht und menschliche Natur. In: Düx G, Marquard O, Ströker E (Hg.) Helmuth Plessner Gesammelte Schriften. Bd. V. Frankfurt a. M.: Suhrkamp. 135–235.

Rawls J (1971) Eine Theorie der Gerechtigkeit. Frankfurt a. M.: Suhrkamp.

Rehbock T (2005) Personsein in Grenzsituationen. Zur Kritik der Ethik medizinischen Handelns. Paderborn: Mentis.

Ricœur P (2005) Das Selbst als ein Anderer. München: Wilhelm Fink.

Scheler M (1927) Der Formalismus in der Ethik und die materiale Wertethik. Halle: Max Niemeyer.

Scheler M (2000) Ordo Amoris. In: Frings MS (Hg.) Max Scheler Schriften aus dem Nachlass. Bd. I: Zur Ethik und Erkenntnistheorie. Bonn: Bouvier. 345–376.

Spaemann R (1989) Glück und Wohlwollen. Versuch über Ethik. Stuttgart: Klett-Cotta.
Tappolet C (2009) Emotionen und die Wahrnehmung von Werten. In: Döring SA (Hg.) Philosophie der Gefühle. Frankfurt a. M.: Suhrkamp. 439 – 462.
Tugendhat E (1998/2001) Über den Tod. In: Ders. Aufsätze 1992 – 2000. Frankfurt a. M.: Suhrkamp. 67 – 90.

Barbara Richartz

Sinn von Krankheit und Motivation zur Genesung

The spiritual meaning of diseases and motivation for recovery

Zusammenfassung: Der Grundgedanke des ärztlichen Handelns besteht in der Linderung oder manchmal sogar der Heilung von Krankheiten. Wir haben es jedoch nicht mit Erkrankungen, sondern mit Menschen und deren Einzelschicksalen zu tun. Deshalb stellt sich im Rahmen einer jeden ärztlichen Tätigkeit immer wieder die Frage nach dem tieferen Sinn einer Krankheit. Im Folgenden möchte ich drei solcher Einzelschicksale, also Patienten mit unterschiedlichen Krankheiten und unterschiedlichen Herangehensweisen an ihre eigenen Erkrankungen vorstellen. Krankheiten können zur Existenzerhellung und zur Eröffnung neuer Lebenshorizonte führen.

Schlüsselwörter: Sinn von Krankheit, Motivation zur Genesung, Existenzerhellung, Horizonterweiterung

Abstract: The basic idea of medical practice is to alleviate or sometimes even cure diseases. However, we are not dealing with diseases, but with people and their individual destinies. Therefore, the question of the deeper meaning of an illness arises again and again in the context of every medical activity. In the following I would like to present three such individual fates, i.e. patients with different illnesses and different approaches to their own illness. Illnesses can lead to a clarification of existence and to the opening of new horizons in life.

Keywords: Meaning of diseases, Recovery, Motivation, clarification of existence, augmented horizons

Einleitung

Erst die Tatsache, krank, gebrechlich oder nicht mehr leistungsfähig zu sein, lässt uns über den Sinn von Krankheit nachdenken. Doch wenn man über Krankheit spricht, muss man zunächst verstehen, was Krankheit ist. Definitionsgemäß ist sie eine Störung der Ordnung, die sich entweder auf Ebene der kleinsten Zellen, der übergeordneten Organe oder der Seele abspielt. Es ist ein Zustand, der von der Normalverfassung abweicht. In der Medizin sprechen wir deshalb auch von den

https://doi.org/10.1515/9783110787153-011

normalen, also physiologischen Abläufen, und den anomalen, also krankhaften oder pathologischen, Abläufen.

Wenn Krankheit eine Störung der Ordnung darstellt, ist die nächste Frage, wie viel Störung eine Ordnung braucht, um nicht mehr funktionieren zu können. Wenn wir uns beispielsweise einen Menschen vorstellen, der verunfallt und sich ein Bein bricht, dann können wir Gesundheit und Krankheit (in diesem Falle den Beinbruch) klar voneinander abgrenzen. Betrachten wir hingegen Laborwerte, dann gibt es eine große Spanne, die sogenannten Referenzbereiche, innerhalb derer der einzelne Laborwert (noch) normal ist. Sollte ein Laborwert jetzt minimal nach oben oder unten von diesem Referenzbereich abweichen, gilt dann dieser Mensch nicht mehr als gesund und ist schon krank? Ähnlich verhält es sich mit Blutdruckwerten, die innerhalb bestimmter Grenzen liegen sollen. Diese Grenzen sind allerdings durch wissenschaftliche Studien definiert. Wenn es neue wissenschaftliche Erkenntnisse gibt, werden genau diese Grenzen angepasst bzw. revidiert. Muss dann auch der Gesundheitszustand der Patienten im Nachhinein revidiert werden?

Wenn wir also von Krankheit und Gesundheit sprechen, haben wir es dann mit einer Polarität – also Krankheit versus Gesundheit – oder mit einem Kontinuum zu tun – also einer Verschlechterung eines Zustandes der langsam in eine Krankheit übergeht? Und was wäre, wenn wir die Polarität aufheben würden, wenn es also keine Krankheit mehr gibt, existiert dann auch keine Gesundheit mehr?

Der menschliche Körper ist auf das Funktionieren ausgerichtet. Schon ein kleiner Defekt (zum Beispiel ein Enzymdefekt) kann das hochkomplizierte und komplexe System ins Wanken bringen. Aus naturwissenschaftlicher Sicht macht dementsprechend Krankheit wenig Sinn. Aus evolutionärer Sicht macht die Krankheit ebenfalls wenig Sinn, denn wenn wir unseren evolutionären Aufgaben nachgekommen sind, nämlich der der Arterhaltung, macht eine langandauernde Erkrankung, ein Gebrechen oder ein Siechtum anschließend keinen Sinn. Wenn die Arterhaltung gesichert ist, könnte der Sterbevorgang unverzüglich beginnen. Im Tierreich findet dies im Übrigen häufig statt. Weibliche Aale – zum Beispiel – versterben, nachdem sie gelaicht haben. Weibliche Spinnen fressen ihre Männchen nach einer erfolgreichen Befruchtung auf und überleben selbst nur noch so lange bis die kleinen Spinnen überlebensfähig sind. Der tiefere Sinn von Krankheit muss also auf einer anderen Ebene, auf einer metaphysischen, zu suchen sein.

Das Paradoxon von Krankheit und Gesundheit

In diesem Zusammenhang habe ich mich gefragt, wie wir uns einen gesunden Menschen vorstellen. Bei meinen Recherchen bin ich auf eine junge Radsportlerin gestoßen: Sie ist 28 Jahre alt, ist 11-fache Weltmeisterin und zweifache Olympiasiegerin. Diese außerordentliche sportliche Karriere funktioniert nur durch tägliche eiserne Disziplin, regelmäßiges körperliches Hochleistungstraining und eine gesunde, auf den Sport ausgerichtete, Ernährung. Scheinbar ein durch und durch gesunder Mensch. Auf dem Höhepunkt ihrer Sportkarriere stürzt die junge Radsportlerin bei einem Training so schwer, dass sie anschließend querschnittsgelähmt ist. Durch ihren eisernen Willen und ihre Disziplin kämpft sie sich zurück in das Leben, das jetzt natürlich anders ist. Erwarten würde man Trauer um das abhandengekommene Leben, vielleicht Wut und Verzweiflung! Anlässlich einer Pressekonferenz sagt sie folgenden Satz mit großer Gelassenheit: „Zum ersten Mal in meinem Leben fühle ich mich richtig frei!" Das Paradoxon von Krankheit kann ein Mensch kaum klarer formulieren. Vorher fährt sie Radrennen, ist in der Spitzengruppe, fährt allen voran – vermeintlich ein freier Mensch. Und exakt in dem Moment, in dem sie sich körperlich nicht mehr frei bewegen kann, fühlt sich ihre Seele zum ersten Mal im Leben frei. Hartwig Wiedebach hat in Anlehnung an Viktor von Weizsäcker einmal gesagt: „Gesundheit ist eine wackelige Brücke über einen Abgrund. Und ihr Einknicken durch Krankheit, Schmerz oder Krisen ist jederzeit möglich und nie ganz zu vermeiden!" (Wiedebach 2016).

Erst das Bewusstsein, dass etwas fehlt, grenzt Krankheit von Gesundheit ab. Hierdurch kann ein Bewusstseinsprozess entstehen, der im positiven Sinne in eine Existenzerhellung führt. Durch die Negativaffekte der Krankheit kann der Mensch/Kranke die tiefsten Einblicke in sein eigenes Ich gewinnen.

Der französische Philosoph Maurice Merleau-Ponty erlitt im Ersten Weltkrieg eine schwere Gehirnverletzung und hatte seither unter erheblichen gesundheitlichen Defiziten zu leiden. Diese Erkrankung hat ihn so verändert, dass er zeitlebens versuchte, den Sinn des Lebens vom Scheitern her zu erfassen. Ähnlich ist es mit der jungen Radsportlerin, die es geschafft hat, ihre Krankheit auf ihren positiven Sinn hin zu lenken. Das, was fehlt/behindert ist, öffnet ihr den Blick auf das, was sein sollte. Krankheit lässt das Leben stillstehen und komplementäre Perspektiven wahrnehmen. Es ist nicht das Paradoxon von Krankheit, sondern das Paradoxon von vermeintlicher Gesundheit.

Die Sprache der Krankheit

Vor einigen Jahren stellte sich ein 60-jährigen Mann in meiner Sprechstunde vor. Bei seiner Erstvorstellung klagte er über ein Engegefühl im Brustkorb, das ihm „den Atem abdrücken würde". Er leitet seit Jahren die IT-Abteilung einer internationalen Firma, ist verheiratet und hat keine Kinder. Sein Lebensmittelpunkt stellt die Firma dar, er ist auf seinen Beruf fixiert und identifiziert sich mit „seiner" Firma. Bei der körperlichen Untersuchung, dem Ruhe-EKG und der Ultraschalluntersuchung des Herzens zeigten sich keine Auffälligkeiten. Bei dem anschließend durchgeführten Belastungs-EKG – einem so genannten Provokationstest – konnten einerseits die Beschwerden reproduziert werden, andererseits zeigten sich EKG-Veränderungen. Beides weist auf eine Durchblutungsstörung des Herzmuskels hin. Daraufhin wurde eine Herzkatheteruntersuchung durchgeführt, eine hochgradige Engstelle im Bereich der Vorderwandarterie diagnostiziert, die in gleicher Sitzung aufgedehnt und mit einem Stent versorgt werden konnte.

Prinzipiell – so sollte man denken – ein großer Erfolg der Kardiologie. Allerdings wurde der Patient nie komplett beschwerdefrei. An einem Tag schienen die Beschwerden besser zu werden, um schon am nächsten Tag wieder vorhanden zu sein. In den nächsten Monaten war er in sich gekehrt, entwickelte eine depressive Stimmungslage mit autoaggressiven Zügen.

Er selbst habe zu viel Stress in seiner Firma und fühle sich den vielschichtigen Aufgaben emotional nicht mehr gewachsen. Er beginnt über seine jahrzehntelang geleistete Arbeit zu reflektieren. Nach seiner Auffassung sei diese nie ausreichend wertgeschätzt worden, insbesondere nicht in der Phase seiner akuten Erkrankung. Nach 6 Monaten stellt er sich erneut in meiner kardiologischen Praxis vor und klagt über eine völlig identische Beschwerdesymptomatik. Auch jetzt wird ein Provokationstest im Sinne eines Belastungs-EKGs durchgeführt. Und erneut kann die Beschwerdesymptomatik reproduziert werden. Es wird wiederum die Indikation zur Herzkatheteruntersuchung gestellt. Und erstaunlicherweise zeigte sich kein mechanisches Hindernis, also keine Engstelle im Bereich der Herzkranzgefäße.

Da in der modernen Medizin ein Kausalitätsdenken besteht, lässt uns dieser Befund fragend zurück. Bei der ersten Herzkatheteruntersuchung war diese Wirkkausalität erfüllt. Die Enge in der Brust, die „die Luft zum Atmen abdrückte", wurde von der mechanischen Engstelle der Herzvorderwandarterie verursacht. Bei der zweiten Herzkatheteruntersuchung konnte diese Wirkkausalität nicht erfüllt werden. Daher versucht man in der Medizin, andere naturwissenschaftliche Erklärungen herbeizuführen. Können Blutdruck oder Puls zu hoch gewesen sein? Oder könnten es eventuell Verengungen der kleinen und kleinsten Herzkranzgefäße sein? Alle konventionellen Therapieansätze haben bei diesem Patienten jedoch nicht zum erwünschten Erfolg geführt. Im Gegenteil: je mehr Medikamente verabreicht und je mehr Untersuchungen durchgeführt wurden, desto mehr haben sich die Symptome meines Patienten verschlechtert. Zum Schluss ließ er sich selbst zu der Aussage hinreißen: „Ich hätte mir gewünscht, wieder ein mechanisches Problem am Herzen zu haben!“

Spätestens an diesem Punkt des Krankheitsverlaufs wird klar, dass eine Krankheit nicht nur behandelt, sondern auch verstanden werden muss. Medizinische Fakten und das Erleben der Beschwerden bzw. der Symptome einer Erkrankung sind nicht synchronisiert. Sie spielen sich auf verschiedenen Erlebnisebenen ab.

Krankheit trifft einen immer unvorbereitet und wirft einen auf sich selbst zurück. Man muss sich mit sich selbst auseinandersetzen. Und dieses Auseinandersetzen erzeugt Wahrheit zu sich selbst und zu seinem Leben. Darum sprechen Patienten von ihrer (eigenen) Krankheit, mit der man am Ende alleine umgehen muss. Krankheit bedeutet Leiden und Leiden erzeugt pathische Fragen nach Ursache und Zweck der eigenen Krankheit! Warum bin ICH krank? Wozu bin ICH krank?

Wahrnehmung und Akzeptanz des Leidens sind für den Patienten wichtig, einerseits durch den Arzt, andererseits durch das persönliche Umfeld. Nur so kann auch der Patient zu einer Akzeptanz seiner Krankheit gelangen. Für unsere Patienten ist es ein basales Bedürfnis, dass eine sprechende beziehungsweise verstehende Medizin durchgeführt wird. Ein Unverständnis für das Leiden – sei es auf organischer oder seelischer Basis – ist mit Sicherheit eine Ursache für die Zunahme chronischer und psychischer Leiden. Das Nichtverstehen und die daraus resultierende Überdiagnostik führen nur zu einer Leidensverstärkung.

Das Leid der Krankheit kann belehrend sein. Durch Leiden kann die Erkenntnis gewonnen werden, dass Krankheit zum Leben gehört. Sie ist eine Konfrontation des eigenen Ichs mit Grenzsituationen.

Bei meinem Patienten können 4 Phasen der Krankheit voneinander abgrenzt werden: In der ersten Phase – der Herzkatheter-Untersuchung – sieht er die Krankheit als etwas an, was behandelt werden muss. In der zweiten, der akuten Phase der Erkrankung, überdeckt der Wille, die Krankheit zu überstehen, sowohl Emotionen als auch Reflexionen. In der sich anschließenden chronischen Phase der Erkrankung ist er gezwungen, zu reflektieren, über den Sinn seiner Krankheit, über den Sinn des Lebens im Allgemeinen und nicht zuletzt auch über den Sinn des eigenen Lebens. Diese Grenzerfahrung mündet – im positiven Sinne – in der vierten Phase der Krankheit, und zwar die Sprache der Krankheit zu verstehen.

Wenn mein Patient sein Leben aufgrund der Krankheit als „Vorlaufen zum Tode“ (Heidegger 1927/1967: 302) zu verstehen beginnt, setzt er sich dadurch vielleicht auf eine Weise mit der „eigentlichen Wahrheit des Daseins“ (ebd.) auseinander, die er sich ohne die Krankheit nicht angeeignet hätte.

Eröffnung neuer Lebenshorizonte

Unter dem Aspekt der Eröffnung neuer Lebenshorizonte möchte ich eine weitere Patientin vorstellen. Sie ist 62 Jahre alt und hat eine unendliche Leidensgeschichte hinter sich. Sie saß bei mir im Wartezimmer, während ich ihre Krankheitsgeschichte studierte.

Mit 18 Jahren wurde die Diagnose „Zystennieren“ gestellt. Diese Diagnose ist nicht behandelbar und führt nach einigen Jahren unweigerlich zum Nierenversagen. Mit 28 Jahren war es dann leider so weit, die Nieren arbeiteten nicht mehr und die Patientin musste an die Dialyse. Im Alter von 30 Jahren heiratete sie und hat ein Jahr später eine gesunde Tochter zur Welt gebracht. Im Alter von 38 Jahren wurde ein Spenderorgan gefunden und sie erhielt eine erfolgreiche Nierentransplantation. Hier könnte die Krankheitsgeschichte eigentlich enden. Das Leiden fing allerdings jetzt erst an.

Nach 12 Jahren glücklicher Ehe verunglückte der Ehemann. In diesem Rahmen erlitt die junge Frau mit 45 Jahren einen schweren Herzinfarkt, musste reanimiert und notfallmäßig operiert werden. Im Alter von 52 Jahren wurde die Diagnose Dickdarmkrebs gestellt. Sie musste operiert werden, sich anschließend einer Chemotherapie und einer Bestrahlung unterziehen. Im weiteren Verlauf kam es durch die Chemotherapie zu einer Verschlechterung der Nierenfunktion, die Niere stellte ihre Arbeit ein. Seit 8 Jahren wird sie jetzt wieder dialysiert.

Diese Krankengeschichte las ich und überlegte, was für ein Patient gleich vor mir stehen würde. Es war eine kleine, zierliche 62-jährige Dame, die mich anlächelte, voller Offenheit und Lebensfreude!

Diese Patientin hatte gezeigt, dass Krankheit neue Lebenshorizonte eröffnen kann. Das Verstehen der Krankheit bedeutet, „ja“ sagen, sie annehmen und als einen Teil des Lebens verstehen. Die Krankheit muss vom Patienten vollzogen, geleistet und gestaltet werden. In Analogie zur Trauer- oder Traumaarbeit gibt es auch eine Krankheitsarbeit. Wie etwa das Fieber, welches die Abwehr stärkt, trägt die Krankheitsarbeit zur Linderung oder Heilung bei. Diese Dame hatte gezeigt, dass man eine Krankheit nicht nur dulden soll, sondern sie auch braucht. Ihre Dialysestation war zu ihrem zweiten Zuhause geworden, dort hatte sie durch die Mitpatienten eine neue Familie gefunden. Darüber hinaus fand bei ihr eine Sensibilisierung für die Schönheit der Natur, eine Sensibilisierung für zwischenmenschliche Kontakte sowie eine Sensibilisierung für traditionelle Werte statt.

Am Leiden können Menschen reifen und wachsen. Leiden bedeutet nicht zwangsläufig Unglück. Diese Patientin hatte gezeigt, dass die Vielzahl der Erkrankungen für sie neue Lebenshorizonte eröffnete. Sie war – trotz oder gerade wegen der vielen Krankheiten – dankbar für das Geschenk des Lebens. Viktor Frankl hat einmal gesagt: „Erst unter den Hammerschlägen des Schicksals ... gewinnt das Leben Form und Gestalt“ (Frankl 1946: 118).

Am Ende bleibt die Frage offen, wie viel Leid und Schmerz ein Mensch ertragen kann. Im Volksmund wird gesagt, dass jedem Menschen nur so viel auferlegt wird wie er auch ertragen kann. Aber warum ertragen manche Menschen ihr Leid oder ihre Krankheit besser als andere. Warum brechen einige Menschen unter der Last des Leidens und der Krankheit zusammen?

Interessant sind in diesem Zusammenhang zwei Fragen an die Patienten:

Was hilft Ihnen, die Krankheit zu ertragen?

Gibt es eine gelingende Krankheit?

In der modernen Gesellschaft sprechen wir von der Resilienz, also dem Vermögen, einmal mehr aufzustehen als hinzufallen. Sind es dann vielleicht die Patienten, die immer wieder „aufstehen“, die auf die Sinnfragen der Krankheit eine positive Antwort haben?

Literatur

Frankl V (1946) Ärztliche Seelsorge. Wien: Deuticke.

Heidegger M (1927/1967) Sein und Zeit. Tübingen: Max Niemeyer.

Wiedebach H (2016) Der pathische Ernst von Krankheit und Gesundheit. Online: https://www.philosophie.ch/blogartikel/highlights/gesundheit/der-pathische-ernst-von-krankheit-und-gesundheit.

Index

https://doi.org/10.1515/9783110787153-012

www.ingramcontent.com/pod-product-compliance
Ingram Content Group UK Ltd.
Pitfield, Milton Keynes, MK11 3LW, UK
UKHW022226051026
15624UKWH00002B/382

9 783110 786873